Community Development Handbook

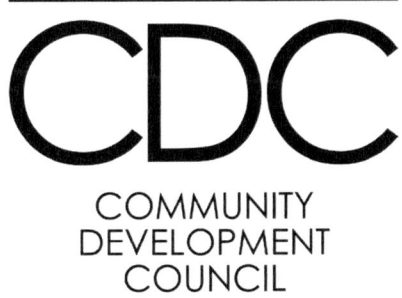

Table of Contents

Foreword 4

Introduction..6
Monieca West

Author Biographies..12

YEAR I

Community and Economic Development Practice 19
Michael John Dougherty & Shelby Fiegel

Community Asset Mapping and Assessments 41
Michael S. Yoder

Community Strategic Visioning and Planning.. 59
Stacey McCullough

Identifying and Developing Stakeholders, Leaders, and Volunteers...................... 78
Lesley Graybeal

Understanding Community Economies 95
Corey Parks & Jamie Gates

YEAR II

Building Entrepreneurial Communities 114
Jeff Standridge & Tiffany Henry

Business Attraction and Site Selection 146
Robert H. Pittman

Business Retention and Expansion 167
Dennis E. Williamson II

Community and Economic Development Finance 183
Toby Rittner

Quality of Place 209
Talicia Richardson & Claire Kolberg

YEAR III

Community Leadership Development 225
Rhonda L. McClellan

Marketing Your Community 246
Amanda Sutt & Valerie Kinney

Measuring Community Progress 270
Rhonda Phillips

Workforce Planning and Development 290
Courtney Taylor & Heather Annulis

Sponsored by

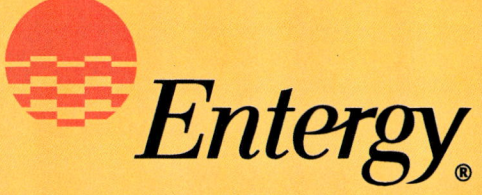

Foreword

Community development facilitates economic development. This concept is the core of what we believe at the Community Development Council (CDC), the governing body of the Community Development Institute (CDI) sites across the nation.

We recognize that every citizen in our communities is a crucial part of community development work. Our goal is to identify community leaders and champions that will lead the charge at the local level and provide them with the skills and strategies they need to make an immediate, positive impact in their communities. At CDI, participants learn how to connect community assets with opportunities, build consensus with local and regional leaders, and sustain the economic development process over time.

How do we do that? We have developed a curriculum that serves as a holistic approach to community and economic development via the *Community Development Handbook*. The primary purpose of this handbook is to serve as the foundation for the training provided at all CDI sites. The handbook's contents drive not only what is taught at CDI, but is the basis for the content of the Professional Community and Economic Developer (PCED) exam, the certification administered by the CDC for graduates of CDI.

The *Community Development Handbook* can also serve a variety of other CED professionals, teachers, students, and those interested in the field of community and economic development as a reference guide and resource. The handbook is composed of diverse topics that make up the umbrella that is community and economic development—but by no means does it cover all subjects that fit within the realm of community and economic development. As we continue to grow and innovate in the field, we recognize there will always be more to learn.

Previous iterations of the current *Community Development Handbook* have served as our core curriculum since CDI's inception in 1987 and were the foundation for the current curriculum. The latest edition of the handbook was based on the CDC's more than 35 years of experience hosting CDI and with the expertise of community and economic development experts who served as authors, contributors, and supporters.

Community and economic development is a rewarding field. Those that choose to operate in the field of CED help develop communities with robust economies, a flourishing quality of life, and diverse and engaged citizen leaders. We hope that you enjoy your journey through CDI and that this handbook serves you in advancing your knowledge of community and economic development.

Community Development Council, May 2021

The Community Development Council (CDC) is a nonprofit organization founded to promote the advancement of standards of competence for community development professionals through accreditation of community development educational programs, professional certification, and the development of community volunteer leaders. Learn more at: www.cdcouncil.com

CDC Board Members, 2021

Ashley Olive, The University of Alabama
Carolyn Motl, PCED, The Motl Group
Christopher Merrett, PhD, Western Illinois University
Courtney Taylor, PhD, PCED, East Mississippi Community College
Frank McCrady, East Montgomery County Improvement District
Gene Stinson, CDC Treasurer, Southern Economic Development Council
Gloria Zacharias, CDC Secretary, Business Oregon
Jerry Miller, Idaho Commerce
Jonathan Dean, PCED, Cleco Power, LLC
Kay Fitzsimons, CDC Chair, Lone Star College
Lisa Taylor, PCED, Durant Industrial Authority
Matthew Twyford, PCED, Arkansas Economic Development Commission
Michael Dougherty, PhD, PCED, West Virginia University
Robin Collins, PCED, City of Eagle
Robert Pittman, PCED, Janus Economics, LLC
Sandy Wittig, Western Illinois University
Shelby Fiegel, PCED, CDC Vice Chair, University of Central Arkansas
Steve Jones, PCED, Arkansas Economic Development Commission
Vic Lafont, PCED, Honorary Advisory Member

CDC Administrative Support Staff, 2021
Matthew Darius, Southern Economic Development Council

Special Thanks

The CDC gives thanks to the sponsors of the *Community Development Handbook*: Entergy, the University of Central Arkansas, and The Motl Group.

The CDC also gives thanks to our handbook editor Liz Russell, graphic designer Kristen Spickard, and Emily Hathcock, PCED, who served on our Editorial Committee.

Introduction

Community developers recognize that an understanding of a community's history is necessary in order to effectively chart its future. The same reasoning applies to organizations such as the Community Development Institute network. This handbook provides its readers with a study in the knowledge and skills needed to be an effective community developer, but it begins with a short remembrance of how it grew from a plan sketched out on a restaurant paper napkin into the national presence it occupies almost four decades later.

The *Community Development Handbook* should be considered a desk reference for those beginning a community development career. Its chapters mirror the curriculum provided by the institutes in the network and is essential to preparation for the Professional Community Economic Developer (PCED) certification.

The practice of community development is informed by the belief that people have the capacity to define their personal and community concerns and develop their solutions. Community developers have the opportunity and responsibility to facilitate this process using best practices grounded in theory. The purpose of this book is to show how this can be accomplished.

Emergence of the Community Development Institute

As with most states in the mid-20th century, Arkansas focused heavily on industrial development, with efforts formalized in 1955 with the creation of the Arkansas Industrial Development Commission, chaired by future governor Winthrop Rockefeller. The state agency sought to diversify Arkansas's economic base by pursuing manufacturing opportunities to supplement those of agriculture. The state realized much success with these efforts, but by the 1980s, leaders began to recognize opportunities beyond these two sectors while also recognizing the importance of creating communities that were capable of taking advantage of them.

The need for community and leadership development was apparent, and this shift in thinking can be traced to Arkansas Power and Light (AP&L), now Entergy Arkansas. AP&L had established a leadership training program for chamber directors and other community leaders in the company's service area, but there was a clear need to expand these efforts. With the leadership of Bill Fountain, Ernest Whitelaw, and Alton Bush, AP&L assembled Arkansas's three major utilities (AP&L, Arkla Gas Company, and Southwestern Bell Telephone Company) and the Arkansas Industrial Development Commission to develop a master plan to build the capacity of communities statewide. The plan had three objectives: reorganize the Arkansas Community Development Society (ACDS) as a professional network for community developers; establish the Community Development Institute (CDI) as a comprehensive source of training with accreditation from the international Community Development Society (CDS); and develop a certification process to elevate the community development profession and enhance the skills of the community development practitioner.

By 1986, ACDS was reorganized with a growing number of members who were in search of a home for the training unit that would become CDI. The University of Central Arkansas (UCA) had begun its economic development outreach in 1982, when Governor Bill Clinton secured legislation that required all public colleges and universities to leverage their capabilities for economic development. These funds, called 10/10 funds, allowed institutions of higher education to develop programs that responded to the development needs of their host communities or to support statewide initiatives. At UCA, this effort was placed in the newly established Office of Corporate Relations under the leadership of Bill Miller.

With only nine months until the doors were to open for the inaugural class, the leadership got to work. Many individuals and organizations contributed to the massive amount of work required to turn concept into reality. Separate committees for general oversight, certification, and curriculum were established, and Dr. Lawson Veasey of UCA joined the effort to develop the frameworks and write the curriculum for each of the three separate years of study. Year I instruction was designed to introduce students to the principles of community development and immerse them in problem-solving situations similar to those most likely to be encountered in their communities. Year II was built around organizing, community engagement, marketing, and strategic planning. Year III focused on putting it all together in a master plan for the community and presenting the plan to the class for feedback.

The inaugural Year I class, held in 1987, hosted 44 students from seven states. In 1988 there were 53 enrolled in Year I, and in 1989—with the first full complement of Years I through III—enrollment totaled 141 students from 15 states. Thirty-three of the original students were the first graduates of the Community Development Institute. While not assured at the time, CDI had the foundation that would serve it well over the next 30-plus years and serve as the springboard for expansion into a national network for community development training, complete with a national certification program.

Certification and Community Development Council

With the Community Development Institute now a reality with a thriving membership base, the leadership turned its attention to certification and accreditation. As an affiliate of the international Community Development Society (CDS), the Arkansas chapter persuaded CDS to establish a certification program in 1989, but the accreditation of CDI was rejected. Because of conflicting views between academics and practitioners, CDS never fully supported certification and would eventually drop it amidst stated concerns of quality assurance, the desire to be inclusive, the fear that certification would create two classes of membership within CDS, and the difficulties of running such a program with volunteers.

When CDS discontinued its certification program in 1995, many people associated with CDI were not surprised and had already begun developing an alternative. The Community Development Council (CDC) was founded in 1995; charter trustees included several people with close ties to CDI. Among them were George McFarland, its first chairman, Jay Robison, Ernest Whitelaw, Ed Toscano, Monieca West, Bill Miller, and Vic Lafont. CDC incorporated in Louisiana with Vic Lafont as its official registered agent and subsequently retained the administrative services of Gene Stinson and the Southern Economic Development Council (SEDC).

The CDC is governed by a 16-member board, which includes representatives from private industry, government, educational institutions, and nonprofit organizations. The board is responsible for assuring the long-term sustainability of the organization. To accomplish this, the Council seeks support from private- and public-sector sponsors and from fees generated by certification and accreditation services. The Council is also responsible for assuring the integrity of certification progress and maintaining a registry of Professional Community and Economic Developers in good standing.

Standardization of Instruction and Handbook

The Community Development Council's sole purpose has always been to promote the practice and application of community development by advancing the highest standards of competence among all practitioners of community and economic development. This includes formal education, training programs, and certification. It also includes a planned approach for the strategic geographic placement of new institutes throughout the United States, approval of common curricula across these institutes, and a certification process that is nationally recognized.

To provide continuity across the Community Development Institute network, CDC works to align all aspects of training and certification. This includes common curricula used by all institutes in the CDI network, a handbook that reinforces the training, and a certification process aligned with the instruction and study materials. Consistency in curricula is important on a number of levels: (1) It assures that practitioners are getting the same base knowledge and that the base includes all critical areas of community development practice. (2) It allows students to accelerate their study by completing sessions at different locations. (3) Testing for certification is more equitable since the certification test is based upon the core curriculum training approved by CDC. While there is a common core of coursework, a level of flexibility allows the institutes to be responsive to local and regional needs.

CDI instruction in Year I includes Community and Economic Development Practice; Community Asset Mapping and Assessments; Community Strategic Visioning and Planning; Identifying and Developing Stakeholders, Leaders, and Volunteers; Understanding Community Economies. Year II includes Building Entrepreneurial Communities; Business Attraction and Site Selection; Business Retention and Expansion; Community and Economic Development Finance; Quality of Place. Year III includes Community Leadership Development; Marketing Your Community; Measuring Community Progress; Workforce Planning and Development.

Entergy Arkansas developed and provided the original community development study guide in the early days of CDI. This was replaced in May 2006 when CDC published the *Community Development Handbook* which is now in its third edition. While the previous edition was more theory oriented, this new edition focuses on helping the practitioner understand how to directly apply abstract concepts to concrete world situations. The *Handbook* addresses all elements of community development, and the chapters correlate with the major topics taught during the three years of CDI.

PCED Certification

The Community Development Council oversees the Professional Community and Economic Developer (PCED) certification program, which is intended for professionals currently involved in the practice of community development who may have a career need for professional credentials. The PCED process involves the identification of core competencies required for effective community development, integration of those competencies into training opportunities, development of supporting study materials, a proctored testing procedure that assesses understanding of how the concepts are applied to community situations, and a method for recertification beyond the initial three-year period.

The PCED certification is delivered in two parts. Part 1 covers content from chapters in this handbook, and Part 2 consists of three case studies in which the applicant is asked to apply knowledge gained from CDI training, this handbook, and their personal work experiences.

To be eligible to sit for the PCED test, the applicant must meet eligibility criteria, pay a fee, and pass a written examination. Eligibility requires that the applicant complete all three years of CDI training from an official CDI site and meet any other requirements determined by the Community Development Council.

The PCED is valid for three years, after which the applicant must apply for recertification and provide evidence of continued professional education, contributions to the profession, and service and participation in community development meetings and programs. A database of people who have been certified is maintained by the Southern Economic Development Council (SEDC), and a network of trained proctors to administer certification testing has been established. Testing is offered at multiple times throughout the year at each training site in the CDC network.

Full information regarding certification can be viewed at www.cdcouncil.com/PCED.htm.

Community Development Institute Network

The Community Development Council achieves its goals through a planned approach for the strategic geographic placement of new institutes so that access to quality training is available throughout the United States.

Since 1987, the Community Development Institute network has grown into a national presence with institutes linked by common goals and curricula that allow students to complete the CDI curriculum by attending one or more programs within the CDI network, commonly known as fast-tracking. There are currently five institutes: CDI Central (University of Central Arkansas, Conway, Arkansas); CDI Midwest (Western Illinois University, Macomb, Illinois); CDI Northwest (Idaho Department of Commerce, Boise, Idaho); CDI Southwest (University of Alabama, Tuscaloosa, Alabama); and CDI Texas (Lone Star College, The Woodlands, Texas). Institutes have been offered in other areas for short periods of time including locations in California, Louisiana, and West Virginia. Efforts to grow the network to provide expanded geographic access are an ongoing goal of CDC.

Community Development Institute and Community Development Council Impact

The Community Development Institute has come a very long way from the 44 people who enrolled in the first class of CDI more than three decades ago. Since then, more than 1,400 community leaders and development practitioners have participated in the Central, Texas, Midwest and Northwest Community Development Institutes. Since its first offering, nearly 300 individuals have received the PCED certification.

Leaders of the Community Development Council and the CDI network understand that there is still work to be done. They recognize the opportunity for growth through organizing and engaging an alumni network and promoting the existing national network through a robust marketing plan customized to target geographic areas. They are also aware of the need to promote training and certification on a national level rather than engaging in regional approaches. This will require that the network consider innovative delivery methods that are fluid and flexible—perhaps a combination of traditional and online delivery. This flexibility will allow the CDI network to continue to be relevant and produce graduates with the desire and skills needed to create quality communities.

The introduction to this handbook is intended to provide history and context for the organization that you are now a part of. CDI and CDC have been blessed with longstanding support from corporate and organizational partners such as the Entergy Corporation, but the heart and soul of both has always been the individuals—the charter organizers, the faculty and staff, the class instructors, and most of all, the students. We wish you well in your endeavors and look forward to your ongoing involvement in and support of the CDI and CDC.

—Monieca West
CDI Inaugural Class of 1987

Author Biographies

Heather Annulis, PhD, CPLP, serves as Director of the School of Interdisciplinary Studies and Professional Development and Professor of Human Capital Development at The University of Southern Mississippi. She holds a doctorate from Southern Miss in International Development with a concentration in Workforce Training and Development. Annulis's research interests include workforce development, creating change readiness, and implementing successful change in organizations through the talents of people. She regularly speaks at regional, national, and international conferences on these subjects. Awards recognizing her professional efforts and research include The Best Published Case Study Award, ROI Institute; Distinguished Professor of e-Learning; Innovator in Workforce Development, Southern Growth Policies Board at the Governor's Association; *Mississippi Business Journal*'s Top 40 Under 40; and most recently, The 2020 Karen Sock Woman of the Year, Lighthouse Business & Professional Women.

Michael Dougherty, PhD, is a Professor and Extension Specialist with West Virginia University. His current research and outreach efforts focus on planning and community development. He has a PhD in Planning and a master's degree in Urban Affairs from Virginia Tech. He serves on the board of trustees of the Community Development Council and on several committees for the National Association of Community Development Extension Professionals. He has worked with local governments and community organizations across the Mountain State for over a quarter century and for the last decade, he has taught planning courses at WVU.

Shelby Fiegel, PCED, is the Director of the University of Central Arkansas Center for Community and Economic Development (CCED) and the Community Development Institute (CDI). She is an Honors graduate of Arkansas State University and holds a degree in Public Relations with minors in Marketing and English. Shelby is a certified Professional Community and Economic Developer (PCED), designated by the Community Development Council, and is a 2016 graduate of CDI. She has also completed the Mid-South Basic Economic Development Course. In 2017, Shelby received the New Professional Award from the Arkansas Community Development Society. She currently serves as the Ex Officio (having previously served as Vice President of Membership and as Vice President of Technology) for the Arkansas Community Development Society, serves on UCA Staff Senate, is a member of the Breakthrough Solutions Advisory Board, Arkansas Economic Developers and Chamber Executives, the Public Relations Society of America (PRSA) and the PRSA Arkansas Chapter. Shelby serves on the Conway Historic District Commission and is an Arkansas Municipal League *City & Town* magazine contributor. She is a graduate of the inaugural class of the Conway Area Leadership Institute (CALI) and is a Certified Strategic Doing Workshop Leader.

Jamie Gates, CCE, is Executive Vice President of the Conway Area Chamber of Commerce and Conway Development Corporation. During his time in city government and private, nonprofit economic development, Gates has led efforts to finance and build more than $100 million in local infrastructure. He is a Certified Chamber Executive and graduate of the Community Development Institute. Gates graduated from the University of Central Arkansas with a degree in Finance.

Lesley Graybeal, PhD, is the Director of Service-Learning and Volunteerism at the University of Central Arkansas in Conway, Arkansas, where she supports partnerships between local nonprofits, faculty members, and students for community-engaged learning and civic engagement. Her research focuses on the impacts of service-learning and experiential learning on nonprofits, faculty, and students, the perspectives and motivations of community partners as educators, and the role of community-generated knowledge in institutions of formal learning. She earned BA and MA degrees in English and a PhD in Social Foundations of Education from the University of Georgia.

Tiffany Henry is the Director of Entrepreneurial Communities at The Conductor, where she empowers entrepreneurs by forming strategic civic partnerships, coordinating rural programming, and leading small business advocacy initiatives. Tiffany holds an MS degree in Psychology from Arkansas Tech University and is a Certified Group Facilitator through the Arkansas Public Administration Consortium.

Valerie Kinney is the Senior Content Marketer at Rock Paper Scissors and has a background rich in all aspects of the content creation process. During her time at Rock Paper Scissors, she has worked with many clients and projects in community and economic development, developing marketing plans, messaging, and collateral for Forward Rabun, Gateway85 Community Improvement District (CID), Gwinnett Habitat for Humanity, and Sugarloaf CID. Valerie is also involved with Rock Paper Scissors' strategic partnership with the Janus Institute for Community & Economic Development and played a key role in the development of Prosperous Places, a resource for sharing knowledge and ideas on how to move communities forward for all interested persons. She holds a bachelor's degree in Mass Communication from Brenau University.

Claire Kolberg is director of The Unexpected and works on special projects surrounding economic and cultural developments. She brings more than 15 years of experience in arts administration and management, production, and operations.

Rhonda McClellan, EdD, holds BA, MEd, MA, and EdD degrees and has taught and coordinated leadership graduate programs in New Mexico, Texas, Vermont, and Arkansas. She currently serves as a full professor in Leadership Studies at the University of Central Arkansas. Her research interests include leader development and integrative community leadership, and she has published in a variety of journals, including *Journal of Leadership Studies, Journal of Higher Education,* and *Journal of Research on Leadership Education.* She has served on the Community Development Institute Advisory Board since 2013 and was awarded the Community Champion by her CDI class. She lives in Arkansas with her husband and four children—Braeden, Dava, Izzy, and Isaac and their Shih-Tzu, Zoe.

Stacey McCullough, PhD, is the Director for Community, Professional & Economic Development with the University of Arkansas System Division of Agriculture Cooperative Extension Service. She oversees programs in leadership, local government, strategic planning and action, economic development, community and regional capacity building, workforce development, program planning and evaluation, and digital learning. Dr. McCullough holds a BBA in Economics from the University of Arkansas at Little Rock and an MA in agricultural and applied economics from the University of Wisconsin–Madison. She has a PhD in Public Policy from the University of Arkansas, where her research focused on local entrepreneurship policy as a rural economic development strategy.

Corey Parks, PCED, is the Vice President of Economic Development for the Conway Area Chamber of Commerce and Conway Development Corporation. Corey earned a Bachelor of Business Administration in Insurance & Risk Management and a Master of Business Administration from the University of Central Arkansas. He is a certified Professional Community and Economic Developer (PCED), designated by the Community Development Council, and a graduate of the Community Development Institute and the University of Oklahoma Economic Development Institute.

Rhonda Phillips, PhD, FAICP, dean and professor at Purdue University, previously served at Arizona State University as professor and director, School of Community Resources and Development and Senior Sustainability Scientist in ASU's Global Institute of Sustainability. A three-time Fulbright award recipient, Rhonda is a planning and development specialist with community quality of life and well-being a focus of her research and outreach activities. Previously, she worked in development at the local and regional levels and held the CED designation for 17 years. She is author of more than 30 books, including Introduction to Community Development, and is editor of two journals, *International Journal of Community Well-Being* and *Local Development & Society.* Rhonda was the first woman to graduate from the Georgia

Institute of Technology with a doctorate in City and Regional Planning. She also holds an MS in Economic Development from the University of Southern Mississippi.

Robert H. Pittman, PhD, PCED, has extensive experience in community and economic development in both the private sector and academia. His economic development and business location consulting assignments have spanned the globe, and he served as an associate professor of Community and Economic Development and Executive Director of the Community Development Institute at the University of Central Arkansas. He is the co-author and editor of the book *Introduction to Community Development*, and he has published more than 50 professional and academic articles in the field. Most recently he founded two organizations to help move communities forward: the Janus Institute and Prosperous Places. He holds a PhD in Economics from Northwestern University and an honorary doctorate of Business from Piedmont College.

Talicia Richardson, PCED, has acquired a wealth of knowledge crossing multiple business disciplines, possessing over 25 years of experience in operations, quality control, and counseling in the industries of hospitality, healthcare, housing and the nonprofit sector. Upon graduation from the Community Development Institute, Talicia earned her certification as Professional Community & Economic Developer (PCED) and moved into the field of community development. As the Executive Director of 64.6 Downtown, Talicia cultivates development through strategic integration of art and culture with community and economics. Talicia holds a BA degree in Sociology from Spelman College and an MS in Counseling from the University of Arkansas in Fayetteville.

Toby Rittner, DFCP, is President and CEO of Council of Development Finance Agencies (CDFA), a national association dedicated to the advancement of development finance concerns and interests. He is a vocal and recognized leader of the development finance industry nationwide and has advised state and federal government leaders, including President Biden and President Obama's Administration Transition Teams. A frequent speaker at local, state, and national conferences and events focused on economic development finance, he is the author of CDFA's highly acclaimed *Practitioner's Guide to Economic Development Finance*. Rittner holds a Bachelor of Arts in Political Science and a Master's of City and Regional Planning degree from The Ohio State University. In 2016 he was awarded the Ohio State University College of Engineering Distinguished Alumnus Award. Rittner is an adjunct faculty member at The Ohio State University and Carnegie Mellon University, teaching planning and finance for sustainable economic development. He is also a Development Finance Certified Professional (DFCP) and has completed the prestigious Oxford University Sustainable Finance Foundation Course.

Jeff D. Standridge, EdD, serves as Managing Director of the Conductor and Co-managing Partner of Cadron Capital Partners. He is an adjunct professor in the College of Business at UCA, where he teaches on the subjects of entrepreneurship, finance, and innovation. Jeff holds the Doctor of Education degree with special work in Leadership and Organizational Development, and a Master of Education with a focus in Adult Education and Human Resource Development. Jeff is the bestselling author of *The Innovator's Field Guide: Accelerators for Entrepreneurs, Innovators, and Change Agents*, and co-author of *Creating Startup Junkies: Building Sustainable Venture Ecosystems in Unexpected Places*.

Amanda Sutt is the CEO and Creative Director at Rock Paper Scissors and oversees the vision and direction of the company while working with her team to develop brands that connect with their clients' audiences and marketing solutions that help clients grow their businesses. Over the years, Amanda has served as Creative Director on a number of projects related to community and economic development, including the City of Duluth, Georgia; Rabun County, Georgia; Community Foundation for Northeast Georgia; United Way of Greater Atlanta; Gateway85 Community Improvement District (CID); Janus Institute for Community & Economic Development; and Sugarloaf CID. Amanda is currently the Vice President of the Janus Institute's board of directors and is a past board member for the Gwinnett Chamber of Commerce. She holds a bachelor's degree from Appalachian State University.

Courtney Taylor, PhD, PCED, serves as the Vice President of Workforce and Economic Development at East Mississippi Community College in Columbus, Mississippi, where she creates and manages degree and non-degree training programs to meet local employer needs. Additionally, Taylor teaches for Troy University and facilitates classes for various Community Development Institutes and previously led the Southeast Community Development Institute. Taylor earned a PhD in Human Capital Development from the University of Southern Mississippi. She has focused much of her career translating needs and opportunities between education, industry, and economic development. Taylor has worked at the forefront of education for the last 14 years, convening diverse stakeholders across academia, industry, and government to develop and implement innovative and robust solutions. Through her collaborative approach to talent creation, Taylor has developed a comprehensive portfolio of training programs aligned with labor market and industry demand. Taylor is also a pioneer in the field of recruitment, where she has implemented a variety of programs designed to engage the next generation of workforce with the STEM economy. Taylor's research interests relate to improving outcomes from training programs and the influence of career counseling on completion.

Monieca West, Director of Federal Programs at the Arkansas Division of Higher Education, manages the Arkansas Career Pathways Initiative and the federal Carl D. Perkins Career and Technical Education program. She is a certified Bridges Out of Poverty trainer and poverty simulation facilitator, an approved trainer for the National Career Development Association *Facilitating Career Development* curriculum, and a certified Strategic Doing workshop facilitator. She has been a board member of the American Indian Center of Arkansas for 30 years, is currently president of the National Association of Career and Technical Education Information, and former president of the international Community Development Society, the Arkansas Community Development Society, and the Community Development Council. She served as Director of Economic Development for AT&T–Arkansas until her retirement in 2000.

Dennis Williamson, PCED, BREC, is currently the Director of Workforce Development and is the EPA Quality Assurance Officer for the Western Arkansas Planning and Development District. He began his career with the district as Economic Development Administrator. Dennis has attended the IEDC business retention and expansion training and holds a Business Retention and Expansion Coordinator designation from Business Retention and Expansion International (BREI). He holds the PCED credential from CDI. He serves as lead for the regional WIOA system business outreach program and as advisor for the City of Van Buren, Arkansas BRE program. He leads a number of communities in the development of more localized programs. Dennis has more than 30 years' experience in key industries with private-sector management and leadership experience. He attended the University of Arkansas and graduated from Liberty University, Summa Cum Laude, with a Bachelor of Science degree in Business.

Michael S. Yoder, PhD, is a geographer who received his doctorate at Louisiana State University in 1994 and his master's at the University of South Carolina in 1989. His early research addressed changing agricultural land-use patterns and related policy in the South Carolina Piedmont, Costa Rica's Nicoya Peninsula, and the Mexican State of Yucatán. He is presently a Research Fellow in the Department of Geography and the Environment at The University of Texas at Austin. From 2008 to 2017 he was Associate Professor of Geography at the University of Central Arkansas, where he served as Director of the Master of Science in Community and Economic Development between 2010 and 2017. Most recently, he has researched suburbanization in mid-sized cities of Mexico and the U.S. Sunbelt, industrial and transport geography in northern Mexico and Texas, and economic development in small cities of Arkansas and south Texas. He is currently writing a book on descriptive case studies of economic development in Texas and Mexico.

YEAR I

Community and Economic Development Practice
Michael John Dougherty & Shelby Fiegel

Community Asset Mapping and Assessments
Michael S. Yoder

Community Strategic Visioning and Planning
Stacey McCullough

Identifying and Developing Stakeholders, Leaders, and Volunteers
Lesley Graybeal

Understanding Community Economies
Corey Parks & Jamie Gates

Community and Economic Development Practice

Michael John Dougherty, PCED
& Shelby Fiegel, PCED

In this chapter, community development is defined as both a process and an outcome, and the relationship between economic development and community development is explained. Participants will learn about the 10-step community development process. The role of the community developer is discussed, especially as it affirms the core values of the discipline. Finally, participants will review a case study and examine a fictional case study in which they must consider steps for effective community development.

Learning Outcomes

- Participants will be introduced to the fundamentals of community development.

- Participants will explore what community development means as both a process and outcome.

- Participants will learn the relationship between economic development and community development.

- Participants will use a community development case study to practice development processes.

Defining Community Development

Community development seems simple, but it is a complex process. The term is comprised of two words—each of which has its own meaning. The first step in understanding community development is to comprehend each of its components. Once those are defined, a common understanding of community development can be established.

Defining the Terms

The word *community* is a noun, often attributive. It has three listed definitions: "a unified body of individuals; a social state, joint ownership, common character or social activity; and society at large" ("Community," n.d.).

The first of these definitions listed has seven subsections and truly outlines the scope of community. Under this definition, community is people with common interests or characteristics. They can be living in a particular area or living together within the larger society or scattered within larger society. They can have a common history or be linked by a common policy or a common location.

The key to this definition is *common*, which should not be surprising since both words come from the same Middle English and Anglo-French root ("Community," n.d.). But what is important is that the locational proximity is not a necessary condition for a community. In other words, communities can be based on place or on interest. This is an important consideration, because too often community development work has focused on just communities of place and ignored communities of interest. This is important as it broadens the scope and potential impact of community development by focusing on what groups different people together, not just that they are grouped together because of their location.

The word *development* is also a noun with three definitions. All three use the verb form associated with the word (*develop*) to define the noun. These definitions are "the act of developing, the state of being developed, or land that has been made usable or is developed" ("Development," n.d.). Meanwhile, the verb *develop* has multiple meanings as both a transitive and intransitive verb. The most applicable definitions appear to be "to cause to unfold gradually" and "to expand by a process of growth" ("Develop," n.d.). Combining the two, a working definition for development is "the act of causing to unfold or grow." Again, it is important to note that this definition may be associated with land (a place) but does not have to be.

Defining the Concept

Combining *community* and *development* into a single term results in a term that most people seem to implicitly understand. Traditional definitions put forth include that of the United Nations (n.d.)—a "process where community members come together to take collective action and generate solutions to common problems"—and the Scottish Community Development Centre (n.d.)—"a process where people come together to take action on what is important to them."

The various organizations in the field

define the term in similar ways. The Community Development Society was founded in 1969 as a national and international network of researchers, practitioners, and policymakers with shared interests. It views community development as a profession that integrates knowledge from many disciplines with theory, research, teaching, and practice as important and interdependent functions that are vital in the public and private sectors (Community Development Society, n.d,).

The National Association of Community Development Extension Professionals formed in 2006 to provide those working in this area within the Cooperative Extension System an organizational home within the Joint Council of Extension Professionals. It defines community development as a "practice-based profession and an academic discipline that promotes participative democracy, sustainable development, rights, equality, economic opportunity and social justice, through the organization, education and empowerment of people within their communities, whether these be of locality, identity or interest, in urban and rural settings" (National Association of Community Development Extension Professional, n.d.). This is based on the definition used by the International Association for Community Development, a global multidisciplinary network (International Association for Community Development, n.d.).

The Community Development Council features a summary of terms under *Resources* on its website. It lists community development as the "act or process of engaging community members to proactively understand and enhance the economic, social, political, environmental, cultural, physical, and educational aspects of a community through the adoption of vision statements, goals, objectives and implementation plans" (Last, 2016, p. 16).

While the details differ in each of these definitions, the core is consistent. Community development is work done for the betterment of a place or group after deliberation by and at the direction of those who will benefit from it.

Two closing notes about community development. The first is that all the formal definitions emphasize the process aspect of community development. Another way to think of community development is as the outcome of all the work done in its name. In other words, the result of community development is community development. The process can be described as "actions," "efforts," "programs," or similar labels. This is analogous to what Dunbar (1972) described as "a series of community improvements which take place over time as a result of common efforts of various groups of people" in his CDS presidential speech. Meanwhile, the outcome can be described as "projects" or "results."

Second, while community development includes housing-related matters, it is much more than that. The notion that housing equals community development may be the result of national-level programs that often commingle the two concepts. The National Community Development Association promotes programs of the U.S. Department of Housing and Urban Development (HUD), the Community Development Block Grant (CDBG), and HOME Investment Partnerships (HOME) programs (National Community Development Association, n.d.). Also, the National Association of Housing and Redevelopment Officers offers training for community revalidation and development professionals which focus on housing topics (National Association of Housing and Redevelopment Officers, n.d.).

Defining Economic Development

The foundation of the Community Development Institute (CDI) is the idea that *community development* facilitates *economic development*, and that success in one area cannot exist without success in the other (or only in extremely rare cases). Community development is the development and creation of assets and resources, whereas economic development can be viewed as the mobilization of those assets and resources. Again, one cannot be successful without the other; they are tied to one another.

A community must find the balance between both areas of development to become a thriving place where people want to "live, work, and play." This section of the chapter will explore the ins and outs of economic development and its role in our communities.

There are many ways to define economic development, but it is primarily recognized as a focus on the monetary aspects of a community. People oftentimes have a predefined idea of what economic development is, moreso than community development. Elected officials tend to tout economic development as purely "job creation" or "community growth." And if you were to ask someone on the street what economic development is, they may think of it in similar terms: job creation, new business development or expansion, or a city's growth in population.

While these conventional ideas of economic development are correct, they only scratch the surface of what economic development entails. There is not a standard definition that is widely accepted for the term *economic development*, but generally it is defined as the process of creating wealth through the mobilization of human, financial, capital, physical, and natural resources to generate marketable goods and services (Last, 2016, p. 20). It includes mobilizing assets and resources to create more and better employment opportunities, an increased standard of living and quality of life, and diversification of a community's local economy (Chadwell, 2019). Economic development encompasses the programs, activities, and policies that seek to improve the economic well-being and quality of life of a community, by creating and/or retaining jobs that facilitate growth and provide a stable tax base.

Economic development should also not be synonymous with community growth (Owen, 2016). Growth, when unplanned, does not always lead to better outcomes. While economic development *can* include community growth, it should only be considered truly successful economic development when that growth is planned.

A good way to think of this concept is to imagine a garden. A planned garden that has been nurtured and thoughtfully developed may include a variety of flowers or vegetables neatly set in rows with no weeds in sight. Yet, a garden where seeds were thrown haphazardly and weeds left unattended may look as robust in terms of "growth" as the planned garden but ultimately would not be viewed in a positive light. The unplanned garden will likely face challenges in the future if left neglected.

Our communities can be thought of along these same lines, but fixing unplanned growth and neglect in our communities is much more difficult and time-consuming than a garden. We must recognize that the best way to move forward is to have a plan in place to mitigate growth issues.

The traditional model of economic development is the "three legged stool" (Chadwell, 2019). The three legs represent: (1) retaining and expanding businesses, (2) recruiting new industries and developing an attraction program, and (3) facilitating the development of small businesses, entrepreneurs, and new business startups. While the three-legged stool can be the base for economic development, in the new global economy economic development has expanded to encompass the areas of workforce development, tourism, leadership development, placemaking, retail, historic preservation, small-scale development, and grow-your-own strategies.

Gone are the days of "build it and they will come." It is essential that community and economic developers and community leaders understand that to be competitive in our current market it takes more than a spec building, cheap land, and/or incentives to entice a new business to move to a community—or even for an established business to decide to expand there. A planned, focused, and holistic approach that combines both community and economic development strategies is needed.

The Relationship between Community Development and Economic Development

What is the relationship between community development and economic development? In reality, "it's complicated" because of the connections between the two activities. The terms, although often used interchangeably, mean different things (Cowart, 2015).

Community development and economic development are sometimes listed as separate efforts, and sometimes they are combined into a single effort. Some places have different departments for each task while other places have them under the same organizational entity. As a result, there are two primary ways to think about this relationship.

In situations where the terms are combined into "community and economic development" or "community economic development," the meaning varies with context. In academic settings, the terms are sometimes used interchangeably to broadly describe all development activities (e.g., Hirschl & McReynolds, 1989). Others see the terms as separate parts of the same process (e.g., Pittman, Pittman, Phillips & Cangelosi, 2009).

Similarly, practitioners utilize the combined term in different ways. The National Association of Counties uses it to describe a multifaceted discussion on development (National Association of Counties, n.d.). Meanwhile, the North Carolina Community Development Initiative describes community economic development as a specific poverty-fighting approach (North Carolina Community Development Initiative, n.d.).

Nevertheless, the concepts have generally retained their own identities. And while there are many ways to define the relationship between community development and economic development, two paradigms are most common.

One way the relationship is typically defined is that community development and economic development are done separately and simultaneously. Under such a system, community development works on issues related to quality of life and is primarily the responsibility of the public sector; economic development works on issues related to income growth and is primarily the responsibility of the private sector. This is the approach taken by the Fort Collins (Colorado) Chamber of Commerce (Fort Collins Works, 2020).

The other way of thinking about the relationship is that community development is foundational. In other words, a place must undertake community development before economic development can occur. This is the point made by the CEO of the Danville-Boyle County Economic Partnership in discussing the roles of each activity (Lassiter, 2015).

The reality is a combination of these different ideas. Some community development—infrastructure—is needed before economic development—provision of good jobs—occurs. But the result of economic development—wealth generation—is necessary to fund community development—quality of life improvements. One way to visualize this is a spring that continues to move in an upward direction. This never-ending cycle builds upon itself with an improvement in one area enabling an improvement in the other area.

How this works in practice will depend on the circumstances of a place. If strong support for economic development already exists, work can begin there before additional community improvements need to be made. In the absence of such a system, community development must be undertaken first to permit successful economic development activities. Future efforts, either community development or economic development, would build upon the previous activity. That is what results in the cycle of continuous improvement—and the confusion about the relationship between community development and economic development.

The Community Development Process

The foundation of community development is that it is defined as both an outcome and a process. The 10-step community development process (Peterson, n.d.) acts as a guide that can be used to identify a scope of work and creates momentum to accomplish a community's economic and community development goals. It is crucial that throughout the process a broad range of citizens are involved to create buy-in and move the process forward.

The 10-step process is as follows and is intended to be cyclical in nature as a community grows and develops:

1. **Begin the process.** The first step in creating change at the community level is to define a process for development and follow that process. Though the community development process is intended for planning at the community level, it can easily be adapted for use in a variety of organizational structures, businesses, or other formal and informal groups. The process begins simply by identifying a group that is in need of assistance.

2. **Engage the community and legitimize the process.** There are multiple ways to engage citizens in a community development process such as public meetings, community-wide surveys, interviews and focus groups, and social media campaigns. When citizens are able to provide suggestions, share their opinions, and have other opportunities to take part in the process they are more likely to support and legitimize it. Consider how you will engage community leaders and make them aware of your planning efforts. Oftentimes in our communities, it is easy for well-intended conversations about our community to disintegrate into nonproductive complaint sessions or personal disagreements. Successful community development occurs when diverse voices join together to have open conversations about their community and tackle challenges to

create a brighter future. One of the most difficult challenges to overcome in our communities is the development of trust between elected officials, community leaders, and citizens. It is essential to create a process of communication that ensures everyone is heard, respected, and supported.

3. **Form an organizational structure.** Forming an organizational structure is an extremely important foundational piece of the community development process. When developing an organizational structure, be intentional about whom you invite to the table. Consider community members from various sectors of the community: public office, chambers of commerce, economic development, education, healthcare, utilities, downtown merchants, businesses (both small and large; local, national, and international), nonprofits, the faith-based community, the arts, and those who are considered community champions. It is also important to think about who your internal and external stakeholders are. A good way to form an organizational structure is to first conduct a stakeholder analysis.

4. **Develop a strategic vision and action plan.** A strategic vision is an overview of where your community wants to be at in a specific time in the future. Depending on the type and duration of the project, your vision can potentially be short- or long-term. The most important part of developing a vision is that all stakeholders in the process agree on the vision and use it as the foundation for the process. Your vision should be aspirational but also achievable. When you have developed a vision that creates buy-in, you can then move forward to develop an action plan. Your action plan should consist of short- and long-term community and economic development goals that focus on the needs of your community as determined by citizens and leaders. These needs can focus on areas such as: education, workforce development, job creation, infrastructure, quality of life and place, downtown development, retail development, housing, poverty, and a host of other community and economic development issues. Finding a balance between goals that can be completed quickly (but also have high impact) and more long-term goals will allow your process to maintain momentum as it moves forward.

5. **Seek feedback and commitment from the community.** When your plan has been developed, go back to citizens you have engaged throughout the process to seek feedback before finalizing it. In completing this step, the community can reengage with the process and continue to develop buy-in. Any last-minute changes or adjustments can also be made to the plan before it is finalized. This also allows for the community and its leadership to commit to the process, which will be significant moving forward.

6. **Publicize the plan.** Your plan is finalized! To spread the word, consider the best communication strategies. Using a combination of communication tools is the best method to spread the word. Host a public unveiling of the plan (and invite key leaders at the local and state level), share with local and state media, print physical copies of the plan and place them in key locations in your community, and share digitally via email, newsletters, city and community websites, and on social media. Word-of-mouth is the number one tool when communicating in your community, so encourage community members to share with their family, friends, and neighbors.

7. **Implement the plan.** The transition between the planning stages of the community development process to the implementation stage can be daunting. It is crucial to begin working on a combination of high-impact short- and long-term goals to maintain momentum. Continue to engage new leaders in the process to achieve your goals.

8. **Evaluate the effort.** Remember that we learn from failure, not success. Ask yourself, "What is working? What is not working?" Make adjustments as needed. Methods to evaluate your efforts include questionnaires, surveys, determining impact and outcomes, and measuring progress made on goals identified in your plan. Personal and group reflection are also good tools for evaluation. This approach would include reviewing the process from each person's unique perspective (including yourself) and sharing opinions on what worked and did not work.

9. **Celebrate your success.** When you complete a goal in your plan, let it be known! To celebrate your success, make sure that those involved in the process know that they are appreciated. Share accomplishments with the public so they are made aware of the good work being done. Determine a communication strategy to spread the word when you achieve a goal or hit a milestone.

10. **Create an ongoing development process.** As stated previously, the community development process is cyclical. As our communities grow and develop, our needs change. Repeat the process as needed.

The Role of a Community Developer

A community developer has always played many different roles. About five decades ago, several attempts were made to define the role. The result was ever-expanding lists but also a constant understanding of what community development work involved.

Cary (1972, p. 36) found "enabler," "encourager," and "facilitator" in a search of the literature and added "educator" and "organizer" to fully encapsulate the work of community developers.

Kelsey (1972, quoted in Austin, 1975) noted that other listed roles including "issue identifier," "leadership developer," "linker," "information provider," "alternative analyzer," "planner," "decision maker," "implementer," "program evaluator," and "provider of rewards and penalties."

Abshier (1973) described it as "impossible" to define the roles. Instead, he proposed classifying roles by functional input in the process or by the level of technical assistance provided.

Where the community developer plays these roles has changed over time. Blakely and Bradshaw (1982) found that community developers had become a resource for institutions, not just individuals and groups. This change came about because the forces that shaped community development changed. They concluded that this new role relationship would require a greater level of preparation and professionalism. Similarly, Shaffer (1990) talked about the need for community developers to set the stage for development activities and help residents understand the development options available. In both cases, these new expected activities align with the facilitation and education roles previously outlined.

More recent research has focused on core competencies rather than specific roles. Gruidl and Hustedde (2015) defined seven competencies for encouraging democratic practice. They described three as foundational and four as functional. The foundational competencies are listening, emotional awareness, and cultural awareness and humility. The functional competencies are public deliberation, facilitation, appreciative inquiry, and empowerment.

One of the resources listed by Gruidl and Hustedde is the Standards Council for Scotland. The most recent version of standards document lists seven general competencies for its term "community learning and development" (CLD Standards Council, 2018):

• Know and understand the community in which we work

• Build and maintain relationships with individuals and groups

• Provide learning and development opportunities in a wide range of contexts

• Facilitate and promote community empowerment

• Organise [sic] and manage resources

- Develop and support collaborative working
- Evaluate and inform practice

Interestingly, a component of the second competency—*build and maintain relationships with individuals and groups*—includes a list of different roles that will need to be played in the work: facilitating, supporting, leading, and advocating. This demonstrates the constancy of the field as these roles are the same as, or similar to, what had been listed in the early inventories of roles for community developers.

Function

The function of a community developer depends on the situation. How community development is defined will determine what someone does under that label. The Federal Reserve Bank of San Francisco described community development as practices and programs that help low-income individuals and communities (Reid, 2011). This is not surprising that many who work as community developers in governmental agencies at the national or state level emphasize the economic and social assistance aspects of community development in their efforts.

Others, as noted previously, view community development as part of or a companion to traditional economic development activities. Their actions could involve garnering public support for a community-wide effort to guiding the community through public works infrastructure improvements. Essentially, they endeavor to create the links in the chain that connect community development and economic development defined by Pittman, Pittman, Phillips, and Cangelosi (2009).

Overall, the function of community developers is viewed as all of this and more. Talmage (2020) stresses the connection between quality of life, community well-being, and community development. Under such an interdisciplinary approach, there is a great deal of overlap between the three activities. As a result, the work of community developers becomes defined in terms of improving the well-being of the community as a whole and the quality of life for the members of the community. Such a description encompasses multiple roles for community developers and multiple purposes for undertaking community development.

Principles

Regardless of what a community developer does, there are professional expectations in how they conduct themselves and undertake their work.

The Hippocratic Oath talks about not doing "harm or injustice" to patients (National Institutes of Health, 2002). This should be considered the base minimum standard for any activity, including community development. More specific to the profession, the Community Development Society created its "Principles of Good Practice" (Community Development Society, n.d., "Principles"):

- Promote active and representative participation toward enabling all community members to meaningfully influence the decisions that affect their lives.

- Engage community members in learning about and understanding community issues, and the economic, social, environmental, political, psychological, and other impacts associated with alternative courses of action.

- Incorporate the diverse interests and cultures of the community in the community development process; and disengage from support of any effort that is likely to adversely affect the disadvantaged members of a community.

- Work actively to enhance the leadership capacity of community members, leaders, and groups within the community.

- Be open to using the full range of action strategies to work toward the long-term sustainability and well-being of the community.

These five concepts provide core guidance for those working in this field. They stress working to ensure broad involvement, participant engagement, diverse ideas and individuals, community capacity building, and a focus on sustainability and well-being.

It is in this context that community developers distinguish their actions as they take a holistic approach to improving circumstances for the people and places they serve.

Ethics and Values

There needs to be a set of values that structure the actions of community developers. Typically, this is done through their ethics system. Ethics refers to a way of thinking and acting. It involves a combination of personal, moral, legal, and social standards. Its function is to determine what is "right" (Rabinowitz, n.d.).

The Community Development Council's summary of terms notes the importance of ethical standards. It discusses them in terms of the professionals who work with community developers, specifically engineers and appraisers. Likewise, it mentions the standards of professional conduct for appraisers and economic developers (Last, 2016).

Likewise, the International Association for Community Development discusses ethics in "Towards Shared International Standards for Community Development

Practice." In the report, the underpinning values of community development are defined as "[c]ommitment to rights, solidarity, democracy, equality, environmental and social justice" (International Association of Community Development, 2018, p. 13). It is also noted these value positions involve applying the ethical standards of practice in context.

The International Economic Development Council, a prominent professional organization for economic developers, has a 12-point code of ethics (International Economic Development Council, 2015). The code stresses matters such as respectfulness, integrity, objectivity, representativeness, transparency, cooperativeness, and equality. It deals with maintaining appropriate confidentiality and abiding by professional principles. It also prohibits sexual harassment and exploiting misfortune.

Likewise, the Community Learning and Development Standards Council of Scotland currently has a 12-part code of ethics for its activities (CLD Standards Council, 2017). Many points of the code are similar, including focusing on the client, empowering constituents, engaging in transparency, cooperating with others, promoting equity, and upholding confidentiality. It expands on these basic principles as it calls for professionals to avoid exposing constituents to harm, to remember the social and ecological context of their actions, to maintain self-awareness, and to keep professional boundaries. It also calls for community developers to improve professional capacity and to undertake self-care.

Finally, community development activities can also serve as a lens through which the ethicalness of other community and economic activities can be viewed. For example, Reed (1999) noted that community business corporations (community-owned firms established to meet local needs) can raise the question of whether it is ethical for profitable businesses to abandon economically disadvantaged places to seek higher profits elsewhere.

Case Study 1
Utilizing the Community Development Process: Kick Start Lonoke

In 2016, the small Delta town of Lonoke, Arkansas began a transparent, respectful conversation that resulted in the creation of a vision for the future with input from citizens in all neighborhoods of the community. Lonoke embarked on a nine-month community development process in partnership with the University of Central Arkansas's Community Development Institute (CDI) and the University of Arkansas Cooperative Extension Service Office of Community and Economic Development to create its strategic blueprint for the future. The community's sense of urgency, passion, and broad base of support from diverse, passionate citizens signaled that Lonoke was ready and willing to plan for the future.

Only 22 miles east of Little Rock, Lonoke is closely linked with the central Arkansas region, though its agricultural base gives it strong ties to eastern Arkansas and the Delta. In June 2016, Lonoke was selected as CDI's Community Development Kick Start community. During the first week of August 2016, the CDI Advanced Year class, a group of experienced community and economic development practitioners, conducted a high-level assessment of Lonoke and provided local leaders with their first impressions and insights on growth opportunities. This was accomplished through a driving tour, online research, data mining, and interviews and focus groups with locals. The Advanced Year assessment served as the catalyst for the first three steps in the community development process: beginning the process, engaging the community, and forming an organizational structure.

Following the CDI Advanced Year experience, the community met monthly to identify key issues and opportunities. Monthly meetings engaged a diverse group of citizens, the attendance of each meeting ranging from 50 to more than 100 community members. The organizational structure of Kick Start Lonoke intentionally involved elected officials, chamber of commerce representation, educational and healthcare representatives, local utilities, business, nonprofit and faith-based leaders, and community organizers. This leadership group was identified as the Executive Committee. This committee also developed a stakeholder analysis and organizational structure, as shown below:

Kick Start Lonoke
Stakeholder Analysis and Organizational Structure

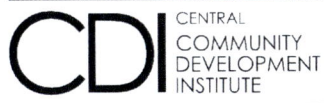
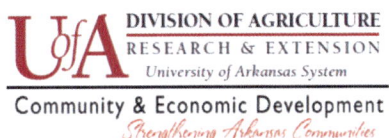

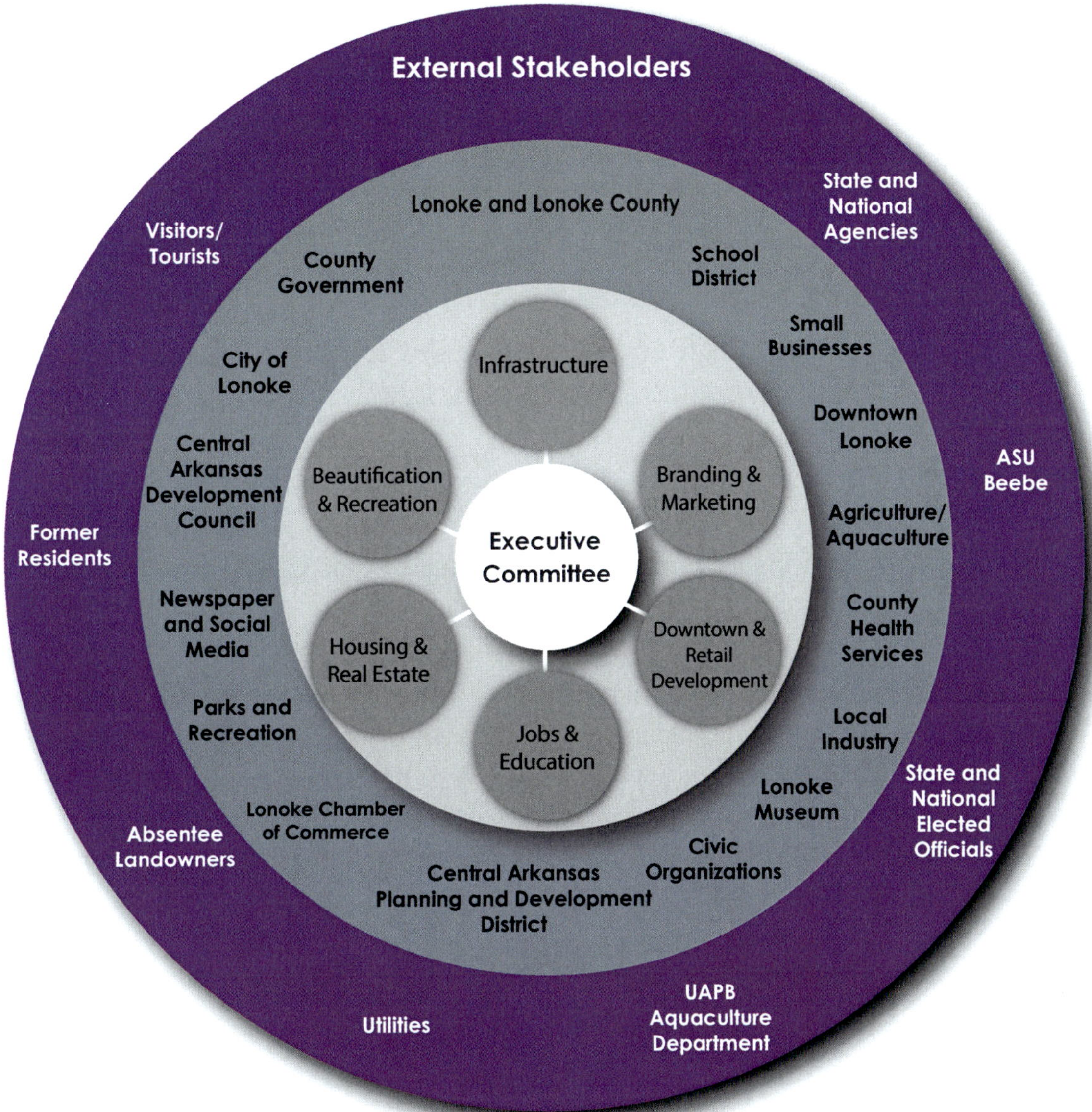

Beyond the Executive Committee, the Kick Start Lonoke process was primarily driven by six Action Teams, composed of citizens interested in moving their community forward. These Action Teams served as conduits for community feedback and commitment. They focused on six areas of improvement: Beautification & Recreation, Downtown & Retail Development, Jobs & Education, Housing & Real Estate, Branding & Marketing, and Infrastructure.

The Executive Committee, with input from the Action Teams and the community, developed a strategic vision for Kick Start:

We envision A VISIBLE, ATTRACTIVE, and CONNECTED Lonoke:

- Kick Start Lonoke envisions a community that is visible to innovative, forward-thinking companies, creative professionals, and families of all ages, when experienced in person or online.
- Kick Start Lonoke envisions a community that is attractive and possesses a mix of skilled labor, residential options, a comprehensive education system, and accessible real estate.
- Kick Start Lonoke envisions a community that is connected to our region and state by economic relationships and logistics, and connected to our neighbors.

The six Action Teams met monthly over a nine-month period to develop short- and long-term community and economic development goals. The process culminated in the unveiling of a five-year strategic action plan in May 2017.

Though Lonoke identified the development and publication of the strategic plan and vision as Kick Start Lonoke, the community decided to launch an implementation phase and rebrand as Lonoke 2022. The rebranding initiative recognized the five-year window beginning in 2017 to achieve the goals of the plan, coinciding with Lonoke's upcoming 150th anniversary in the year 2022.

Since launching of its plan in 2017, Lonoke has made great strides and achieved successes such as:

- launching the first farmers' market in Lonoke (Fishtown Market)

- development and implementation of a new community brand

- the "Connecting Lonoke" study developed by Mississippi State University students, which created vignettes for pilot projects focusing on Two Prairie Bayou

- State Highway 31 corridor enhancements

- Downtown Lonoke public space

- Lonoke Community Center expansion and outdoor recreation

- Lonoke Ballpark enhancements and a greenway recreational network

- recreational trails now occupy the former railroad right-of-way

- new businesses are bringing experiences that the town has not previously known

- acceptance into Main Street Arkansas's Downtown Network program

Throughout its community development process, Lonoke has evaluated its efforts, made adjustments as necessary, and celebrated its successes to create a successful, ongoing development process. By following the community development process, Lonoke has been able to leverage incremental change to develop a brighter future. To learn more about Lonoke 2022, visit http://www.lonoke2022.wordpress.com.

Case Study 2
The City of Linkin

Put your skills to the test with a fictional case study! Think carefully about the lessons you've learned in this chapter to recommend next steps for the fictitious community of Linkin.

Your first step is to read the information about Linkin below. Then, determine a course of action. What would you recommend be done?

The City of Linkin's new mayor has identified a corridor in its downtown area that is in serious need of revitalization. The mayor has approached the Linkin Downtown Partnership and Linkin Area Chamber of Commerce about initiating a visioning process to revitalize this corridor.

Significant public and private investment has been made in the downtown area over the past 10 years. However, this stretch of street and property, referred to as the Smith Street corridor, continues to see little investment, resulting in blight and underutilization. The corridor has a thriving private liberal arts college on one end and the downtown business district on the other. It is also next to a low-income residential area. Many homes and lots in this residential area are owned by one or more out-of-state individuals who have inherited property from deceased relatives. Commercial activity is limited to a bail bondsman and a dry cleaner.

Consider other information about the community and the corridor:

- A potential brownfield site (old scrap metal yard) is located on a property in the Smith Street corridor. No one is sure what cleanup would cost, and no one has spoken with the property owners about their plans for the future. This site has become almost invisible to the locals who drive past it every day, but there is a feeling among local leaders that it is driving away investment.

- Antiquated utilities in the area pose an additional cost to its redevelopment. The local utility provider, Linkin Corp, is city-owned and manages all utilities except natural gas. Linkin Corp will make up to $5 million in utility improvements per year within the city, but other areas of the community are competing for this limited investment.

- In addition to the private liberal arts college, the City of Linkin is also home to a four-year university.

- Recently, many small developers have begun to restore old homes in the nearby historic district, but none of their investment has trickled over to the Smith Street Corridor. In a recent meeting with the mayor, the developers expressed concern that there was no plan for revitalizing the area and there had been limited public investment that might make private investment more attractive.

Consider the following questions as you think through this scenario:

- What would be the first step you would take to initiate a visioning and planning process for the City of Linkin?

- Who are the stakeholders you would want to include in this process and why? How would you include these various groups?

- What would be your strategy as you move throughout the visioning and development process?

- What are some of the key issues that you anticipate you would need to address during the revitalization effort?

As you think through these questions, remember the relationship between community development and economic development, the 10-step community development process, and your role as a community developer. Using the lessons learned in this chapter will enable you to formulate a course of action for the City of Linkin (Whitehead, 2019).

References

Abshier, G.S. (1973). Roles of the professional community developer. *Journal of the Community Development Society, 4*(1) 109–114. DOI: 10.1080/00103829.1973.10877496

Blakely E.J. &. Bradshaw, T.K. (1982). New roles for community developers in rural growth communities. *Journal of the Community Development Society, 13*(2): 101–120. DOI: 10.1080/15575330.1982.9987154

Cary, L.J. (1972). Roles of the professional community developer. *Community Development, 3*(2), 36–41. DOI: 10.1080/15575330.1972.9674816

Chadwell, J. (2019, July 29–August 2). *Introduction to economic development* [Conference session]. Community Development Institute, Conway, AR, United States.

CLD Standards Council for Scotland. (2017). *A code of ethics for community learning and development.* https://cldstandardscouncil.org.uk/wp-content/uploads/Code_of_Ethics_2017.pdf

CLD Standards Council for Scotland. (2018). *The competent practitioner framework: Using the CLD competencies to reflect, develop and progress.* https://cldstandardscouncil.org.uk/wp-content/uploads/CompetentPractitionerFramework.pdf

Community. (n.d.) *Merriam-Webster.* (Online dictionary) https://www.merriam-webster.com/dictionary

Community Development Society. (n.d.). About CDS. https://www.comm-dev.org/about

Community Development Society (n.d.). Principles of good practice. https://www.comm-dev.org/about/principles-of-good-practice

Cowart, W.C. (2015). *Community development vs. economic development.* LinkedIn. https://www.linkedin.com/pulse/community-development-vs-economic-w-chad-cowart-rla/ (Accessed Sept. 23, 2020)

Develop. (n.d.) *Merriam-Webster.* (Online dictionary) https://www.merriam-webster.com/dictionary

Development. (n.d.) *Merriam-Webster.* (Online dictionary) https://www.merriam-webster.com/dictionary

Dunbar, J.O. (1972). The bedrock of community development, *Journal of the Community Development Society, 3*(2), 42–53. DOI: 10.1080/15575330.1972.9674817

Fort Collins Works. (n.d.). *Community development vesus ecnomic development.* http://fortcollinsworks.com/community-development-versus-economic-development/

Gruidl, J. & Hustedde R. (2015). Towards a robust democracy: The core competencies critical to community developers. *Community Development*, 46(3), 279–293. DOI: 10.1080/15575330.2015.1028082

Hirschl, T.A. & McReynolds, S.A. (1989). Service employment and rural community economic development. *Journal of the Community Development Society*, 20(2), 15–30. DOI: 10.1080/15575338909489980

International Association for Community Development. (n.d.). Home page. https://www.iacdglobal.org/

International Association of Community Development. (2018). *Toward shared international standards for community development practice.* https://www.iacdglobal.org/wp-content/uploads/2018/06/IACD-Standards-Guidance-May-2018_Web.pdf

International Economic Development Council. (2015). International Economic Development Council Code of Ethics. https://www.iedconline.org/index.php?submenu=CodeofEthics&src=pages&ref=code-of-ethics

Kelsey, G. (1972). Community resource development process. A Great Plains Community Development Publication, New Mexico State University Cooperative Extension Service. Cited in Austin, J.K. (1975). Initial contact approaches for community resource development with small rural communities. [Thesis, New Mexico State University]. https://files.eric.ed.gov/fulltext/ED106011.pdf

Lassiter, J. (2015). Economic development or community development? Develop Danville. https://www.developdanville.com/news/details/lassiter-economic-development-or-community-development

Last, G. (2016, January 5). *Summary of economic development terms* (3rd ed.). https://www.edpbestpractices.com/resources/economic-development-terms-acronyms

National Association of Community Development Extension Professionals. (n.d.). What is community development? https://nacdep.memberclicks.net/what-is-community-development-

National Association of Counties. (n.d.). Community & economic development. https://www.naco.org/topics/community-economic-development

National Association of Housing and Redevelopment Officers. (n.d.) Certification and training. https://www.nahro.org/certification-training/

National Community Development Association. (n.d.). Overview. https://ncdaonline.org/overview/

National Institutes of Health, History of Medicine Division, National Library of

Medicine. (2002). North, M. (Trans). Greek medicine: "I swear by Apollo physician …": Greek medicine from the gods to Galen. https://www.nlm.nih.gov/hmd/greek/greek_oath.html

North Carolina Community Development Initiative. (n.d.). What is community economic development. (Accessed Sept. 23, 2020).

Owen, I. (2016, August 1–5). *Introduction to economic development* [Conference session]. Community Development Institute, Conway, AR, United States.

Peterson, M. (n.d.). Ten step community development process. Community Development Council. http://www.cdcouncil.com/documents/TenStepCommunityDevProcess.pdf

Pittman, R. Pittman, E., Phillips, R. & Cangelosi, J. (2009). The community and economic development chain: Validating the links between processes and outcomes. *Community Development, 40*(1), 80–93. DOI: 10.1080/15575330902918956

Rabinowitz, P. (n.d.). Ethical Issues in community interventions. In *Community Tool Box*. Center for Community Health and Development, University of Kansas. https://ctb.ku.edu/en/table-of-contents/analyze/choose-and-adapt-community-interventions/ethical-issues/main

Reed, D. (1999). Ethics, community development and not-for-profit business: The case of New Dawn Enterprises. *International Journal of Social Economics, 216*(5), 660–673.

Reid, C. (2011). CI notebook. *Community Investments: Federal Reserve Bank of San Francisco, 23*(1), i. https://www.frbsf.org/community-development/files/CI_FullIssue_Spring2011.pdf

Scottish Community Development Centre. (n.d.). What is community development? https://www.scdc.org.uk/who/what-is-community-development

Shaffer, R. (1990). Building economically viable communities: A role for community developers. *Journal of the Community Development Society, 21*(2), 74–87, DOI: 10.1080/15575339009489962

Talmage, C.A. (2020). Community development, quality of life, and community well-being: Three fields ripe with opportunities for future research and practice. *Community Development Practice, 24*(1), Article 4. https://egrove.olemiss.edu/cdpractice/vol24/iss1/

United Nations. (n.d.). Uniterm: Community development. https://web.archive.org/web/20140714225617/http://unterm.un.org/DGAACS/unterm.nsf/8fa942046ff7601c-85256983007ca4d8/526c2eaba978f007852569fd00036819?OpenDocument

Whitehead, A. (2019). *Case study: City of Linkin*. University of Central Arkansas.

Community Asset Mapping and Assessments

Michael S. Yoder, PhD

This session emphasizes the importance of undertaking a community assessment early in the development process, that is, prior to strategic planning. Participants learn the SWOT (Strengths, Weaknesses, Opportunities, Threats) approach and how to garner both qualitative and quantitative information about their community. The session explains the need to conduct assessments, how they fit into the overall development process, and best practices in assessing communities. It includes examples of community assessments and their use. Participants will also learn the difference between an asset-based and need-based approach to development. A perspective that emphasizes assets, rather than deficiencies, creates more momentum for positive change. Participants become familiar with the different types of assets utilized in communities and learn techniques to identify assets in their own communities.

Learning Outcomes

- Participants will discuss identification of strengths, weaknesses, opportunities, threats, and other factors that influence the community development process and outcomes.

- Participants will review how and why community assessments are conducted.

- Participants will explore data collection methods, best practices, and how assessment fits in to the overall community effort.

The Nature of Community Assessments

Communities need to actively evaluate their place in the ever-changing global economic system. Commercial investment, migration, and threats of the global pandemic will be with us for the unforeseeable future and will reshuffle the deck in terms of the impacts of global economic, health, and climate trends on localities, and vice versa. In short, each community's preparedness for changing global trends depends on planning. A community assessment is a useful project for keeping abreast of a community's potential for development and resilience; the assessment process enables a given community to meet a breadth of objectives that such planning identifies.

A community can range in scale from a neighborhood to an entire city or town. Perhaps an individual neighborhood could benefit from enhanced attention toward a particular need that affects quality of life, such as a shortage of recreational amenities or youth unemployment. Likewise, a city overall might face such focused needs. A community might also wish to examine a broader array of issues subsumed in economic development than the need for new employment opportunities, such as an improvement in community health delivery, the reinvigoration of downtown, or the enhancement of the city-wide park system. Local stakeholders need to identify whether a community assessment is desirable, and if so, the issues to focus upon (Heaven, 2010). If a community desires to create a strategic plan, a marketing plan to attract investment, or a plan of action to solve a specific problem or set of problems, a community assessment is a prerequisite (Vincent, 2015b). Community assessments can empower communities to carry out actions if they enable the community to match capabilities with resources (Smathers & Lobb, 2014). In short, they are an integral part of the process of community development and improving quality of life (Haines, 2015).

If a community desires to create a strategic plan for problem solving, it is not enough to tackle symptoms; it is necessary to identify and address root causes of the problems. For example, the objective of attracting needed employment may be hindered by some underlying cause of the lack of good jobs. The solving of such problems is an example of a needs-based assessment (Haines, 2015). The community assessment, then, should focus on workforce quality first and foremost, and the conditions of other assets like transportation systems or the availability of land secondarily. A comprehensive community assessment will reveal the feature or features of the community that are most appropriately addressed. That said, the most successful community assessments are "asset-based," emphasizing how a community's strengths should be capitalized upon for the benefit of the community and its economic development. By doing that, and by prioritizing citizen participation in the process, the community's assets will become more apparent to a greater number of people, maximizing feelings of greater ownership and belonging on the part of the participants in the assessment (Haines, 2015; Vincent, 2015b).

The position of the Community Development Institute and Community Development Council is that a comprehensive, asset-based approach is most helpful for enabling stakeholders to transform a community. The community assessment initiative needs to be planned carefully ahead of time, monitored during its implementation, and assessed after the fact. Furthermore, the community assessment should be revisited fairly regularly after it is completed (Heaven, 2010). The major directors of the assessment need to be like-minded so that the assessment follows a coherent path. To take the point further, successful outcomes emanating from a community assessment require conditions commonly referred to as a positive "community spirit," a "can-do attitude," "pro-business attitudes," and the like (Vincent, 2015b, p. 192). Case Study 1 illustrates the need for local decision makers responsible for issues related to community development, including the production of a successful community assessment, to be on the same page. (Case Study 1).

Community Definitions

Community assessments can be applied to a variety of "communities." A community is usually a spatial entity, such as a neighborhood or a municipality, whose boundaries can be defined fairly precisely. It can also include adjacent municipalities, Census-designated places, and adjacent rural areas that function together because of their inseparable proximity. The designation of a spatially delineated community, however, is not always the focus of an assessment. Thus, the definition can be more flexible than that. It can also be "a collection of people with common, social, economic, political, or other interest regardless of residency" (Vincent, 2015a, p. 103). Those carrying out the different parts of the community assessment should be representative of the diversity of the community, including age, race and ethnicity, gender, and perspectives on the issues, to the extent possible (Heaven, 2010).

Sometimes the effort to create an appropriate definition of a community will prompt the initiators of an assessment to include nearby assets that are not located within the legal boundaries but nonetheless impact upon a community's success. For example, an interstate highway a few miles away from—but not within—a given city's boundaries can nonetheless provide opportunities (Vincent, 2015b). Others who define a community will attempt to include adjacent municipalities. Examples of such inclusion of two or more municipalities defining a community are Minneapolis and St. Paul, Minnesota; Memphis, Tennessee, and West Memphis, Arkansas; and Texarkana, Arkansas and Texas (Vincent, 2015b). It may or may not be appropriate to include another contiguous municipality or Census-designated place. Several community stakeholders in the Texarkana case indicate that because that metropolitan area straddles a state line, it is quite difficult for the two municipalities to think of themselves as one community in their day-to-day functioning. Case Study 2 provides a summary of my own research of two communities of Arkansas with unclear—and often incompatible—definitions of community. (See Case Study 2.)

Data Collection for the Assessment

Data collection is a process that encompasses different options and involves multiple steps.

- The first step is to determine what the assessment will focus upon, followed by the gathering of data that already exists, such as academic studies, news articles, prior assessments by local governments and other organizations, Census data, and other public records (Heaven, 2010; Smathers & Lobb, 2014).

- Commonly the second step is to gather data through "listening sessions and public forums" (Heaven, 2010).

- Third, the process should include interviews. There are different types of interviewing, each with its own advantages and disadvantages, including face-to-face, telephone, and group discussions. Each type can range to varying degrees from structured to semistructured to open-ended. Generally, the interviews of individuals can effectively be the most open-ended.

- Typically, a fourth phase includes focus group interviews or group discussions. These group forums can be structured or semistructured in terms of the questions asked or the topics covered.

- The fifth step is typically direct observation, and participant observation when possible. In that case, those carrying out the community assessment will conduct what is in effect fieldwork to directly observe the phenomenon or phenomena focused upon in the assessment.

- An optional sixth step involves broadly distributed surveys. Whatever instrument is used should be pilot tested ahead of time (Smathers & Lobb, 2014). The advantages and disadvantages of each of the interview types, focus group sessions, and surveys are discussed in the asset mapping and SWOT analysis sections below.

- The seventh step is to develop a final report that includes an executive summary, a description of the methods used, and details about the strengths of a community and an acknowledgment of limitations to overcome (Smathers & Lobb, 2014). (See Case Study 3.)

Asset Mapping

Asset mapping is a data collection technique that emphasizes the community's strengths rather than focusing on community shortcomings, disadvantages, or problems to be solved (Heaven, 2010). It differs from a needs-based assessment, an exercise in directly addressing a specific problem that may need a plan for solving it. The purpose of the asset-based approach to community assessment is to identify the positive attributes of a municipality or neighborhood that can be built upon in the community development process. Surely any weaknesses of a community are revealed during asset mapping, and efforts can then be made to remedy them (Green, 2015). However, an asset-based approach is designed and needed for positive community transformation. The process emphasizes the identification of assets within the community itself rather than features of the area that are not directly in the community and therefore not able to be directly altered by the community. The latter approach ensures that the community focuses on what it can improve upon and rejects the notion that outside assets should be relied upon. The mapping of assets enables the community to better understand which are within the boundaries of the community and which are external (Baird & Peterson, 2020; Human Services Commission, 2013). Generally, the smaller the scale of community under consideration, the more likely asset mapping will be centered on a specific project or theme (Green, 2015).

Once the community's territory is defined and its strengths—institutions such as schools and libraries, associations of citizens, medical facilities, commercial establishments, government facilities, influential individuals, and amenities like parks—are identified, these features can literally be mapped to show their actual locations. But the "mapping" process is also somewhat metaphorical in that it diagrams the connections between valuable features of the community that are regarded as assets. The geographic mapping helps stakeholders think of their community as a "case study" area, which directs attention on the most appropriate resources to build upon. Local histories and their physical landscape features and cultural resources are important to include, and these are spatially mappable. Assets include capabilities, such as skills, leadership proficiencies, and workplace experience ranging from art to repair to customer service, and medical care (Green, 2015). Furthermore, asset mapping can be utilized for community development initiatives that are specific, such as youth programs, or more general, such as economic expansion (Baird & Peterson, 2020; Human Services Commission, 2013).

Careful consideration must be given to the ways in which the information gathered will be used in asset mapping. How will resources be allocated for the greatest good, in light of what is learned from asset mapping, to enhance community and economic development? To produce a successful asset-based community assessment, not only is it necessary to identify the methods to be used to carry it out; furthermore, the people and data necessary to carry it out must be identified, and tasks must be delegated. Generally, the most knowledgeable people to bring on board include heads of organizations, social clubs, elected officials, and members of local academic institutions (Human Services Commission, 2013).

One of the challenges of asset mapping of economic capabilities is that people in a community spend money outside the community, referred to as leakage, while money comes into the local economy from other areas. Therefore, it is important to include in the mapping process representatives of those sectors of the economy that involve leakage and inflows of spending, such as different retail sectors. Likewise, some assets, while not economically tangible, need to be inventoried, including networking capabilities of a community, institutions, community services, and potential public meeting spaces that might otherwise be overlooked (Green, 2015).

Community assets are wide ranging and therefore valuable to a wide range of citizens. Among the broad categories of community assets are the skills and talents of the workforce and community leaders, the ability of a community to form effective partnerships (*political capital*); social organizations such as organizations, clubs, and churches (*social capital*); the natural setting, built environment infrastructure and architectural features (*physical capital*); the overall economy or availability of *financial capital* for investment; and the health of the citizens and the society, including racial or ethnic harmony. Each community has its own mix of assets, and the results of asset mapping in each will therefore be different (Haines, 2015).

Haines (2015, p. 48) provides a useful breakdown of physical, human, and social capital, which overlap and determine the quality of life of a community:

- **Physical capital** is immobile. Examples include buildings, a downtown or central business district, physical landscape features, transportation systems and infrastructure, education institutions at all levels, utility infrastructure, and industrial parks. Their creation, maintenance, and upgrades involve both private and public investment.

- **Human capital** is mobile and transformable. It includes the "skills, talents, and knowledge of community members." Young people matter as much as those of employment age or older. Human capital can change as people move in or move out of a community—or result from education, training, the gaining of new skills, and other building of capacity. Leadership skills and artistic talent are as important as the jobs skill level.

- **Social capital** includes networks between individuals, groups, and organizations. It includes shared goals that bind a community in meaningful ways that distinguish each community. Different forms of social capital can be formal (including organizations and clubs that undertake community service) and informal (relationships that are of a more personal or familial nature). As Case Study 1 illustrates, social capital, especially the positive relationships necessary to meet challenges, can transcend the community and involve, for example, elected officials whose jurisdiction includes the community in question.

Green (2015, pp. 214–215) lays out a series of steps to be taken and methods to utilize in asset mapping. First, the community should clearly define the goals and expectations of what is to be accomplished. These can be as specific as one issue, such as public health or expansion of a particular social service for the poor, or they can be as broad and comprehensive as attracting outside investment for economic development. Second, stakeholders should define as precisely as possible the territory of the community, which can range from an individual neighborhood to an entire municipality. The definition of individual neighborhoods can be imprecise in comparison to an entire municipality. Usually neighborhood-level asset mapping involves a specific issue, while the city-wide version includes an array of conditions. Third, the methods to be employed for mapping of assets need to be determined. This step can include combining of two or more tools as reviewing existing documents and news articles, open-ended interviews, focus group interviews, and surveys. Each of these techniques has its advantages and disadvantages, and if three are used, a technique referred to as triangulation can enhance greatly the accuracy of the information gathered. Triangulation can be thought of as "checks and balances" whereby the results of one technique can be verified or validated by one or two other methods (Yoder, 2016).

The most common survey methods are face-to-face interviews, mail or web-based surveys, telephone surveys, and group-administered surveys (Green, 2015).

1. Face-to-face surveys usually result in the best response rate and can accommodate nuance and greater detail than a standard printed or online survey with fixed questions. The process can take longer, however, and the person(s) carrying out the surveys should be well trained in this technique.

2. Mail surveys are shorter in length and easier for the persons participating in the survey, but they nonetheless suffer

from lower response rates than other techniques.

3. Web-based surveys, using platforms such as SurveyMonkey, create better response rates but require access to email addresses.

4. Phone surveys produce higher response rates than the web-based version though not as high as interviewing people face-to-face.

5. Group-administered surveys require assembling a meeting and are most feasible when surveying social groups, citizens groups, or clubs. They offer the advantage of quickly accessing a number of people at one time, they are inexpensive to carry out, and can include visual information, such as asset mapping, on the fly (North Dakota, 2019; Green, 2015). The people attending the meeting, however, may not be representative of the neighborhood or overall community (Green, 2015).

I have participated in an asset mapping exercise that involved the collection of background data and news articles, one-on-one (face-to-face) interviews, and group interviews, and I find this arrangement the most preferable because it lends itself to triangulation and includes open-ended discussion where nuance and details can be included.

SWOT Analysis

The SWOT analysis is a useful tool in community assessment and can reveal ways to affect change. SWOT is an acronym for *Strengths, Weaknesses, Opportunities, and Threats*. The concept of the SWOT analysis began within companies and social organizations as a means of assessing their entities' strengths and weaknesses and identifying changes for improvement. However, communities overall can effectively utilize the concept at a much larger scale—for individual neighborhoods or entire cities, their organizations, governing entities, and nongovernmental institutions. Strengths and weaknesses lie within the control of the community, while opportunities and threats are usually external conditions and therefore not under the direct control of the community (Renault, 2018). The SWOT analysis is a useful tool in strategic planning—one of the objectives of community assessments—as well as the creation of a community's marketing plan for attracting new residents and investment (Vincent, 2015a). The ideal application of a SWOT analysis is to emphasize the positive features of a community to build upon (internal strengths and external opportunities) while taking into account the challenges that need to be overcome and addressed (internal weaknesses and external threats) in the community development process (Renault, 2018).

Val Renault (2018) provides useful guidelines for carrying out and utilizing a SWOT analysis. First, those who carry out the analysis need to make a list of the factors that are internal to the community (strengths and weaknesses)—and avoid being overly modest. Among those elements that are internal to the community and appropriate to consider are skills and abilities, physical (immobile) assets, economic conditions, organizations and their activities, the functioning of vital local government (police, fire, utilities) and the community's image. These factors should be considered both from the point of view of the community itself and the perspectives of outsiders, as best as these can be identified. The identification and cataloging of these elements is most efficiently carried out through focus group discussions, community open meetings, interviews of key informants—and secondarily through surveys, given that what is desired is an array of perspectives on the community's strengths and weaknesses (Vincent, 2015a). The results can also produce new ways of utilizing the community's strengths (for example, turning a reservoir that is the source of a community's water into a recreation area). Likewise, a simultaneous focus on weaknesses can reveal areas that need work and improvements in leadership. The process of pondering weaknesses can better enable a community to reverse or even eliminate them (Vincent, 2015b).

Finally, an examination of opportunities and threats, which are external to the community and not under the community's control, is equally useful. Communities can make good use of opportunities and can mitigate potential or real threats over which they would otherwise lack control. The key is to plan for resiliency. Examples include broad economic upswings or downturns, weather and climate, natural disasters, pandemics or other health trends, and geopolitical events such as the terror attacks of 2001. To illustrate, the destruction of the World Trade Center led to an aversion to skyscraper occupancy in central business districts in large cities, which provided an opportunity for suburban communities and their development of office parks (Vincent, 2015b). My own research of international bridges linking Mexico and Texas revealed that the construction of the Anzalduas International Bridge, located on the far west side of McAllen, Texas and administered by the McAllen International Bridge System, provided a benefit to the adjoining city of Mission, Texas, and alleviated traffic bottlenecks in McAllen and communities to the east. Prior to the bridge's opening, Mission had lacked such convenient access to an international bridge that linked to Reynosa, Tamaulipas, Mexico. Thus, the management of one city's threat (McAllen's traffic) became an opportunity for commerce next door (Mission).

Likewise, the establishment of Southwest Florida International Airport (RSW) in 1983 in a rural portion of Lee County southeast of Fort Myers and operated by the county's port authority is an opportunity in the form of enhanced airport access for the nearby cities of Naples and Marco Island. Case Study

4 illustrates some of the uncertainties of transportation assets (Case Study 4). It remains to be seen whether communities that ultimately manage the COVID-19 pandemic relatively well can turn that global threat into a local strength by highlighting their effective leadership.

Final Thoughts

Asset-based community assessments and the mapping of those assets produce awareness of the positive features of the community; as a result, those resources can be better utilized for the community's transformation. The process of examining such resources in detail will lead to a greater awareness of how to utilize them to enhance community connections and subsequent community development. It also expands awareness of the utility of the positive features and resources of the community (Human Services Commission, 2013). A comprehensive plan is a highly regarded product of the knowledge gained from community assessments, asset mapping, and SWOT analyses. A SWOT analysis and asset mapping can be accomplished simultaneously; these different tools are not necessarily discrete and can be complementary (Flora & Flora, 2020). I have observed that in the community assessment process, it is common for participants to refer to other communities' initiatives that they believe might work in their own community. This is a helpful exercise that may very well enrich the final report or strategic plan. It requires extra work during the information-gathering stage but can be well worth the effort. Examples might be Complete Streets initiatives to accommodate more transportation options than automobiles, or traffic circles (roundabouts) that enhance traffic flow by streamlining intersections of two or more streets. Form-based urban planning, employed in some communities around the country, can allow for variations from strict zoning laws on a case-by-case basis to include a mix of residential and commercial land uses, which can invigorate the life of a block or an entire neighborhood. In this type of borrowing of concepts, good ideas can and do diffuse throughout the country.

As of the writing of this chapter, the COVID-19 pandemic has resulted in lockdowns in order to properly isolate citizens. As a result, public meetings otherwise carried out in person are now occurring virtually, through internet technology that utilizes Zoom and similar meeting platforms. Ecommerce has grown during the pandemic while retail establishments, especially those deemed "nonessential," struggle to keep socially distanced foot traffic flowing through their doors (Reese, 2020). The general belief of the majority of community and business leaders is that, while some businesses in the retail and restaurant sectors of local economies will close, most other activities will return to normal once a vaccine has been widely distributed and new cases of the virus shrink significantly or vanish altogether. A common thought among analysts of retail economies holds that the community nature of retailing—including social interaction, face-to-face contact, the tactile delights of browsing in shops, and personalized services—will enable much of the local retail economy to survive (Reese, 2020).

Many of the components of community assessment, asset mapping, and SWOT analysis that involve face-to-face, in-person communication, community meetings, focus group interviews, and the like will need to be carried out virtually in the short and medium terms. Furthermore, educational institutions at all levels will continue to change their systems of teaching as they become resilient to the present and future pandemics. At present, the technologies to handle community forums are improving, though not every citizen has equal access to computers and Wi-Fi. In many households, multiple persons compete for the usage of computer hardware and internet connections, and until these become more universally available, community assessment processes overall will face challenges.

It is not yet known how the community assessment process will be altered now that a pandemic has upended so much about the way people relate and communicate. News stories abound regarding the difficulties of transitioning students at all levels to online learning. Likewise, it is reasonable to assume that focus groups, open community meetings, and even face-to-face interviewing and its usefulness will be impacted. Furthermore, with lockdowns, crowd avoidance, and strict social distancing guidelines, community assets such as festivals, concerts, sports events, and cinema are already impacted strongly, forcing communities to address ways to facilitate social distancing whilst maintaining economic activity. This uncertainty is expected to continue well past the mass distribution of a COVID-19 vaccine ("The 90 Percent Economy, Revisited," 2020). Thus, some of the threats and opportunities of the SWOT analysis are rapidly being redefined. Community assessments involve the identification of ways of catapulting the community based on assets but also on acknowledging the problems or negative elements of a community's milieu and turning those things into positive aspects of a community. How can communities accomplish this goal in the midst and aftermath of COVID-19? Do communities simply "ride it out," or do they seize the challenge and reinvent the community assessment process to confront the pandemic and its alterations to ways of doing the community's business? As communities confront these uncertainties, they will undoubtedly be forced to solve many of them through trial and error.

Case Study 1
The Need for Consensus among Stakeholders: School Reopening during COVID-19

Education is an important part of community development—and can be an important theme in community assessments. Given their importance to society and the ways they can heighten emotions and debate, education initiatives, such as decisions related to the proper reopening of schools during the COVID-19 pandemic, require consensus. This principle applies to many areas of community development and is reflected not only in policy itself but also community assessment. Favorable political capital is an essential ingredient of reaction to the pandemic.

In the summer of 2020, New Mexico Governor Michelle Lujan Grisham established clear guidelines for schools to reopen during the Coronavirus pandemic, while the State of Texas had not yet done so by the beginning of the school year. Lujan Grisham's order allowed public schools without outbreaks to accommodate students at 50% capacity with strict oversight by the New Mexico Public Education Department. Private schools, which are not subject to such oversight, are limited by the state to 25% capacity (Hayes, 2020). The Texas state government, by contrast, decentralized decision making about school reopening to the school districts themselves, offering no clear guidelines as to how districts would work with local health departments (M. Gutierrez, address to Seguin ISD faculty and staff, August 5, 2020).

Under the American federal system, decision making over community development issues of an emergency nature is decentralized, leading to difficulties in establishing clear consensus. In contrast, Denmark, a country with a unitary political system, has successfully reopened schools under a carefully crafted policy involving input from teachers' unions, local school authorities, and parents' organizations. Denmark's Minister of Education, Pernille Rosenkrantz-Theil, explained on the CNN show "GPS," hosted by Fareed Zakaria, on August 16, 2020, that Danish schools had already reopened by early August with students in smaller groups than normal—around 25—in classrooms and hallways, and only come into contact with other members of the small groups; they see no other students. This consensus-based strategy allows for easily managed social distancing as well as contact tracing. Constant assessment of the arrangement means that conditions can be changed if necessary.

Minister Rosenkrantz-Theil mentioned that a strong cooperation of this type cannot be invented on the fly but is part of Danish civic culture (Zakaria, 2020). Thus, it might be difficult for communities in the U.S. to replicate the Danish model. This, then, requires strong and consistent leadership from state officials, as is the case in New Mexico, to operate schools in the era of the pandemic. The principle of this kind of organized collaboration applies to virtually all aspects of community development.

Case Study 2
Should Adjoining Settlements be Viewed as One Community?
Two Examples of Contested Definitions of "Community" in Arkansas

Batesville, Arkansas (population 10,700) and the adjoining community of Southside (population 3,550) comprise the Batesville Micropolitan Statistical Area in Independence County, in the eastern foothills of the Ozark Mountains. In the research I conducted in the two communities, based largely on open-ended interviews, I found quite a lot of ill will between the two. Prior to Southside's incorporation in 2014, the previously unincorporated community frequently rejected efforts by Batesville to annex it. (In Arkansas, annexation can be carried out if the city council of the city undertaking the annexation votes in favor of doing so, regardless of the desires of those in the area under consideration However, most municipal governments strongly prefer the will of the people in both the existing city and the target community.)

The main reasons cited in interviews of business owners of both communities indicated that the primary objection pertained to the prospect of higher property taxes, even though Southside residents had relied on Batesville to provide utilities and waste disposal and lacked a municipal police force.

Batesville pursued annexation to broaden its own tax base. The negativity between the two communities led to the rapidity of Southside's incorporation to prevent annexation. Southside's incorporation in 2014 meant that the new municipality had to construct a city hall and create departments. Ironically, another rural area adjacent to Batesville's eastern city limits desires to be annexed by the city for the sake of improvement of police protection and provision of water and trash collection. Batesville is presently not interested in such annexation, because the costs of providing services to an area whose houses are spread out would not be recouped by taxes or fees.

In the west-central part of the state, Arkadelphia (population 10,650) and the adjoining small municipality of Caddo Valley (population 600) have an interesting history related to both annexation and consolidation. In Arkansas, consolidation requires that both communities in question carry out a favorable vote. Both communities are located on Interstate I-30 in the foothills of the Ouachita Mountains. The interstate, competed in the early 1970s, plays an interesting role in this story of questionable definition of community. Prior to the interstate's completion, the citizens of Caddo Valley, then unincorporated, desired to be annexed by Arkadelphia, given that the latter was relied upon to provide water, trash collection, and other services. The citizens of Arkadelphia, however, viewed the annexation of Caddo Valley as a financial liability, similar to Batesville's regard for the rural area adjacent to its east side.

Upon completion of the interstate, an exit was constructed near downtown Arkadelphia, and another at Caddo Valley. Caddo Valley then incorporated in 1974. Immediately, several motels and restaurants opened in Caddo Valley, thereby enhancing the new municipality's tax base. In 2009, city officials of Arkadelphia proposed consolidation with Caddo Valley, to take advantage of the latter's increased sales and lodging tax intakes. A majority of the voters of Caddo Valley rejected the idea while a majority of those of Arkadelphia supported it. This reversal in the relationship between the two adjoining communities—and their inability to reach consensus—suggest that the two communities should be viewed as separate.

Case Study 3
A Community Assessment in Heber Springs, Arkansas

The Community Development Institute (CDI) Central, in conjunction with the Center for Community and Economic Development (CCED)—both based at the University of Central Arkansas—offers a fourth-year advanced course for graduates of the three-year CDI program. The Advanced Year is an intensive applied course whose acceptance process is selective. In 2015, the Kick Start team worked in the community of Heber Springs, Arkansas. It consisted of seven students, all of whom had community development experience, and an instructor, a professional community developer based in the Office of Community and Economic Development within the University of Arkansas System Division of Agriculture, Research, and Extension. In effect, the team carried out the initial steps of a community assessment based on asset mapping blended with a SWOT analysis, in accordance with the Breakthrough Solutions model of the U of A System Office of Community and Economic Development. The primary purpose of the Kick Start is to introduce leaders in a given community to the benefits of—and guidelines for—conducting out a community assessment utilizing asset mapping, so that they are equipped to carry out a project themselves. Secondarily, the students who attend the fourth-year experience are able to apply the principles and understand in greater detail, through hands-on engagement, the concepts they learned in the CDI program (Peterson, 2015).

The Kick Start Program occurred during the first week of August 2015. The initial steps included online research about the community, including its strengths and weaknesses, by the student participants. The marketing of the community and its assets was a topic of particular importance to Heber Springs's leaders and business community. They desired to build further on its established tourism industry, and to attract additional investment by local businesses and potential outside businesses looking to start or open a facility in Heber Springs, whether retail, hospitality, or manufacturing. The site visit included a meeting of stakeholders to identify further concerns and desires of the community. The student participants worked with these stakeholders to derive a set of recommendations for further action that were presented to an open community forum on the last day. Among the topics covered were:

- the best ways Heber Springs could compete with other tourist destinations and extend the short tourism season to one that is year-round;

- the enhancement of downtown to draw new business and foot traffic;

- the retention of young citizens who tend to emigrate upon completion of school; and

- workforce development to make the community viable for manufacturing or high-skill services.

The administration of the UCA Center for Community and Economic Development has periodically followed up with the main identified stakeholders to assist the community in furthering its community assessment (Peterson, 2015).

Case Study 4
The Transportation Riddle

Asset mapping and the identification of strengths and opportunities often place at or near the top of the list transportation systems, including highway infrastructure, rail lines, canals, coastal ports, and airports. The universal conventional wisdom is that the more developed the transportation system, the more advantaged is a given community. Some of the features of the transportation system, however, can be elusive and counterintuitive. An ongoing study I am carrying out of small cities of Arkansas and south Texas has revealed some transportation riddles. These involve communities located along an interstate highway or a major or secondary rail line who are unable to capitalize on such presumed assets to attract investment in activities that generate employment.

The city of Forrest City (population 14,480) is located in eastern Arkansas, adjacent to Interstate 40 and just 42 miles from Memphis, a major transportation hub for trucking, rail, air cargo, and barges. Yet Forrest City has seen its manufacturing and distribution base stagnate since the 1990s in spite of that proximity. Ironically, Harrison, Arkansas (population 13,087), located in north central Arkansas in the Ozark Region, is connected by two-lane highways to the east, west and south; the only four-lane highway leads north. Despite this, Federal Express Freight, which carries large cargo by 18-wheelers, is headquartered in Harrison. Uvalde, Texas, a city of 16,181 (2018) and the core of a micropolitan region comprised of the county of the same name, occupies a favorable position on U.S. Highway 90, roughly midway between San Antonio and the border twin cities of Del Rio and Ciudad Acuña. Union Pacific Railroad (UP) has a secondary line that skirts the city's north side, and yet only one facility in the city has a small siding that currently links to the rail line. A company that mines construction materials, referred to as aggregates, links to the rail line by a siding eleven miles east of the city. UP makes pickups of gravel and asphalt and drops off empty cars about twice a month. Thus, given its limited use, it is difficult for local community leaders to boast about the UP line as an asset.

In contrast, Gonzales, Texas (population 7,200 in 2018) is located at the junction of the two-lane U.S. Highway 90 Alternate and U.S. Highway 183, 73 miles east of San Antonio, 135 miles west of Houston, and 18 miles south of Interstate 10. The city is served by a short-line railroad, the Texas Gonzales and Northern (TXGN) Railway, that links to the main east–west UP line between San Antonio and Houston, and has been able to capitalize on its rail linkage. TXGN has created a sizable intermodal center immediately north of Gonzales that handles aggregates and other construction materials, sand for hydraulic fracturing in the Eagle Ford Shale region, and storage, repair, and recycling of railcars and locomotives.

My takeaway from these case studies is that a favorable transportation connection alone is usually a necessary but not automatically strong community asset. Other factors come into play, including available and trained workforce, well-established activities in the community and its immediate vicinity, and the right kind of proximity to larger cities.

References

Baird, L. & Peterson, M. (2020). *Introduction to community asset mapping.* Center for Court Innovation. https://www.courtinnovation.org/sites/default/files/documents/asset_mapping.pdf

Flora, J. & Flora, C. (2020). *Community capitals framework model.* P3 Communities. https://www.p3communities.com/about-us/community-capitals-framework-model/

Green, G.P. (2015). Community asset mapping and surveys. In R. Phillips & R. Pittman (Eds.), *Community development handbook* (2nd ed., pp. 213–224). Routledge.

Haines, A. (2015). Asset-based community development. In R. Phillips & R. Pittman (Eds.). *Community development handbook* (2nd ed., pp. 45–56). Routledge.

Hayes, P. (2020, September 5). Public schools and private schools to reopen at different capacities. KOB News. https://www.kob.com/albuquerque-news/public-schools-and-private-schools-to-reopen-at-different-capacities/5852666/

Heaven, C. (2010). Developing a plan for assessing local needs and resources. In Community Tool Box. Center for Community Health and Development, University of Kansas. https://ctb.ku.edu/en/table-of-contents/assessment/assessing-community-needs-and-resources/develop-a-plan/main.

Human Services Commission. (2013, October 30). An introduction to community asset mapping. County of Santa Barbara. https://www.countyofsb.org/ceo/asset.c/400

Muñoz, M. (2020 August 29). NADBank has exceeded expectations, says Rep. Hurd. *Rio Grande Guardian*. https://riograndeguardian.com/podcast-nadbank-has-exceeded-expectations-says-rep-hurd/.

North Dakota Department of Health. (2019). Community assessments. In *Vision to action: Sexual violence and intimate partner violence prevention toolkit* (pp. 57–78). https://www.ndhealth.gov/injury/ND_Prevention_Tool_Kit/docs/Community_Assessment.pdf.

Peterson, M. (2015). *Community development Kick Start report: Heber Springs*. Center for Community and Economic Development & University of Arkansas Division of Agriculture Research and Extension.

Reese, S. (2020, September 8). Integrating retail online/offline experiences in the "new normal." *Multichannel Merchant*. https://multichannelmerchant.com/blog/integrating-retail-online-offline-experiences-in-the-new-normal/.

Renault, V. (2018). SWOT analysis: Strengths, weaknesses, opportunities, and threats. In *Community Tool Box*. Center for Community Health and Development, University of Kansas. https://ctb.ku.edu/en/table-of-contents/assessment/assessing-community-needs-and-resources/swot-analysis/main.

Smathers, C. & Lobb, J. (2014). *Community assessment*. OhioLine, The Ohio State University. https://ohioline.osu.edu/factsheet/CDFS-7

The 90 percent economy, revisited. (2020, September 19). *The Economist* 436 (9212), 67–68.

Vincent, J.W. II. (2015a). Community development practice. In R. Phillips & R. Pittman (Eds.), *Community development handbook* (2nd ed., pp. 103–121). Routledge.

Vincent, J.W. II (2015b). Community development assessments." In R. Phillips & R. Pittman (Eds.), *Community development handbook* (2nd ed., pp. 190–212). Routledge.

Yoder, M.S. (2015.) The sprawling of small cities of Arkansas: The case for sustainable urban planning. *The Arkansas Journal of Social Change and Public Service.* University of Arkansas at Little Rock, Bowen School of Law. https://ualr.edu/socialchange/2015/05/17/the-sprawling-of-small-cities-of-arkansas-the-case-for-sustainable-urban-planning/

Yoder, M.S. (2016.) Cargo transport infrastructure and urban regional development: The Fort Smith Metropolitan Area. *Urbana*, 17, 14–31. https://www.urbanauapp.org/wp-content/uploads/Yoder16.pdf

Zakaria, F. (Host). (2020, August 16). GPS (Global Public Square) [TV. CNN. https://www.cnn.com/videos/tv/2020/08/16/exp-gps-0816-danish-education-minister-on-reopening-schools.cnn

Community Strategic Visioning and Planning

Stacey McCullough, PhD

This session describes a powerful approach to harnessing change in a community: strategic visioning and planning. First, the difference between visioning and planning is defined, and participants learn the steps to implementing a strategic visioning and planning process. Next, the role of the facilitator in the process is outlined. Examples of community visions, goals, and objectives are provided. Finally, participants learn of ways to move into implementation to ensure that the process leads to measurable outcomes.

Learning Outcomes

- Participants will learn the definition of visioning.

- Participants will understand strategic planning and discuss the process.

- Participants will explore the steps to implement a visioning and strategic planning process.

- Participants will discuss the role of the community developer/facilitator in the process.

- Participants will study examples of community mission statements, vision, goals, and objectives.

- Participants will review some of the challenges communities face as they go through the visioning and planning process, and ways these challenges can be addressed.

Communities become what they are based on decisions made and actions taken by people over a long period of time, whether planned or not. A lack of planning will force a community into a reactive, rather than proactive, position. Investments in infrastructure or activities that aren't valued by community members—or are irrelevant in a changing world—may not achieve desired results. Strategic visioning and planning lay the foundation for intentional actions to shape a community's future. While events may occur that change that trajectory, having a vision and plan in place can help a community overcome adversity and identify new opportunities.

While many communities begin a process because they are struggling, it is equally important for those that are thriving. This is in part because forces and trends that shape a community's well-being, such as demographics and technology, change over time. Investing in the time and effort to monitor these changes and consider how they may impact the community's efforts to achieve its vision can improve its chance for success. Although it may be necessary to change plans to adapt to changing circumstances, the process of community visioning and planning provides valuable information that can inform those changes and ensure the community continues to move forward to its desired future.

Community Visioning

Visioning is the process by which members of a community come to a shared understanding about what they want for the future (Center for Rural Pennsylvania, 2006; Lachapelle, Emery & Hays, 2010; Miner & McDermand, 2003; Okubo, 2000). To be effective, the process should include and engage people who reflect the diversity of the community's residents, businesses, elected officials, local institutions, and other stakeholders (Center for Rural Pennsylvania, 2006; Lachapelle Emery & Hays, 2010; Okubo, 2000). A typical process would include one or more facilitated events where residents work in small groups to identify key assets, strengths, opportunities, and their dreams for the future (Center for Rural Pennsylvania, 2006; Miner & McDermand, 2003). The leadership team overseeing the process reviews these, identifies common themes, and combines them into a single statement. This draft vision is shared back with facilitators and other key stakeholders involved in the visioning process for feedback and modification. The end result is a statement, sometimes accompanied by a graphic or brand, that is understood and shared by community members, broad enough to encompass diverse perspectives, inspiring, easy to communicate, and allows the community to adapt to a rapidly changing world (Nagy & Fawcett, n.d.; Okubo, 2000).

While more common in organizational strategic planning, a mission statement is sometimes developed as part of the community strategic planning and visioning process. Whereas the vision statement describes a community's desired future, the mission statement captures the underlying foundation and values of the community now. It provides the context through which the vision will be achieved.

Sometimes the vision statement is composed in a way that includes elements of the community's mission and vision. Exhibit A provides examples of community vision and mission statements.

Exhibit A. Community Vision and Mission Examples

Vision—Berryville, Arkansas

Berryville is a safe and economically stable, sustainable, and diverse community that retains its rich heritage, its natural beauty, and its sense of place.

Vision—Historic Downtown Cedar Hill, Texas

We envision a Historic Downtown Cedar Hill that preserves its distinctive charm and fosters complementary growth; where unique shops, services, dining, cultural attractions, and living opportunities attract visitors and residents to live and work in our community in a safe, friendly, and walkable environment with connections to other parts of the city.

Vision—Broomfield, Colorado

A city and county of diverse neighborhoods that inspire identity and unity; where its culture of excellence, leadership, self-determination, and innovation is nurtured and practiced; and where its businesses thrive and its citizens of all ages are proud to live.

Vision and Mission—Fauquier County, Virginia

Vision Statement: Fauquier County is a thriving community that honors its natural and cultural resources, agricultural heritage and rural landscape while building a sustainable economy and promoting outstanding services and growth within defined service districts.

Mission Statement: Working within the theme of "Progress with Reverence for Heritage" and with a strong commitment to the accomplishment of meaningful improvements to the efficient, effective, and open conduct of the County government, and to the public health, safety, and welfare and educational opportunities, the Fauquier County Board of Supervisors seeks, within the bounds of fiscal integrity, to preserve the physical beauty, historical heritage and environmental quality of the county while ensuring that population growth and development is a positive force on the general welfare of the community.

Strategic Planning

Strategic planning is the process of developing a blueprint or road map for achieving a community's vision (Miner & McDermand, 2003). Because of this connection, communities often create or update their vision as part of a strategic planning process. Like visioning, effective strategic planning involves people representing all aspects of the community. The final product outlines the steps identified by community members as necessary to reach that vision. It includes specific goals, objectives, strategies, and actions that lead to desired outcomes as well as lay out a process for future decision making. Strategic planning is most effective when viewed as an ongoing process (Center for Rural Pennsylvania, 2006; Miner & McDermand, 2003). While a large-scale planning process may only occur every three to five years, a community's strategic plan should be a living document in which progress is monitored and adjustments are made on a regular basis.

Community development researchers and practitioners have used a variety of models for guiding communities through the strategic visioning and planning process since the 1960s (Center for Rural Pennsylvania, 2006; Okubo, 2000). Exhibit B provides an example of major steps followed in a typical visioning and planning process.

Exhibit B. Example of Strategic Visioning and Planning Steps

- Gather information from citizens and stakeholders and secondary data sources to assess the community's current strengths and weaknesses.

- Review internal and external conditions and trends that will impact the community's future.

- Draft and solicit feedback to finalize a community vision.

- Identify community and economic priorities and goals.

- Consider strategies to achieve goals and solicit community and stakeholder feedback.

- Develop an action plan that details the strategies and actions that will be implemented to achieve goals.

While the specific steps and methods used may vary, most strategic planning processes used today share a number of common elements:

- identification of individuals to provide leadership and support for the visioning and planning process, as well as implementation

- engagement of people who reflect the diversity of the community's residents, businesses, elected officials, local institutions, and other stakeholders throughout the process

- compilation of data to inform the process and evaluate the process

- priorities, goals, and action plans, detailed and linked together

- evaluation of progress toward reaching priorities and goals, as well as the process itself

- celebrations of progress and success

Leadership and Support for the Process

The launch of a strategic visioning and planning process is often initiated by local leaders who recognize that dreams for the future don't typically just happen. However, the visioning and planning process will likely include multiple levels of leadership (Center for Rural Pennsylvania, 2006). Most processes begin with the establishment of a steering committee or coordinating body that will oversee the process and keep things moving forward (Miner & McDermand, 2003; Okubo, 2000). This team should include leadership from all sectors and interests within the community who are willing to commit to seeing the process through and are able to work well with others. Members may be added to this team over time, particularly as the community moves from visioning to action planning and implementation. Specific activities of this team include:

- determine the steps and timeline for the planning process;

- secure resources needed to support implementation of the planning process; and

- create and implement a communications plan to share information about the process to community members and encourage involvement

Creating opportunities for other members of the community to assume leadership roles in the strategic visioning and planning process can be helpful in facilitating buy-in, ensuring that things get done, and cultivating a leadership pipeline for the future. Examples include inviting individuals to serve on subcommittees formed to carry out tasks associated with the planning process that are of interest to them, asking them to contribute to parts of the process where they have expertise or access to needed resources, providing them with tools (fliers, social media posts, etc.) to help spread the word about events and developments, or asking them to host or assist with a particular event or task. Follow up by publicly acknowledging these contributions and showing appreciation. Consider escalating "asks" to individuals demonstrating enthusiasm and effectiveness in assuming roles. This will be key to sustaining efforts to achieve the community's vision over time. For additional information, see the chapter "Identifying and Developing Stakeholders, Leaders, and Volunteers" in this handbook.

While not required, many communities decide to bring in an outside facilitator to help guide the process. Assistance is often available from state economic development agencies, community engagement or cooperative extension service arms of universities, planning and development districts, utility companies and rural electric cooperatives, nonprofit organizations, and private consulting firms.

Engaging a facilitator can be helpful in multiple ways (Hinz, n.d.). First, the leadership team may lack the expertise, experience, or time to develop and implement the planning process. Second, an outsider may "see" things people in the community do not. For example, the facilitator may notice sectors of the community not represented on the leadership team or observe untapped assets within the community. Third, an external facilitator may have ideas for alternative ways of tackling elements of the planning process and overcoming challenges faced throughout the process. Fourth, the facilitator may have knowledge of and access to additional resources that can benefit the community in its efforts. Finally, a trained external facilitator can create a neutral or unbiased atmosphere and move the group forward when dealing with difficult or controversial issues.

There can be disadvantages to using an external facilitator as well (Hinz, n.d.). First, they may charge for their services, which could be cost-prohibitive for the community. It may also require extra time so the facilitator can become familiar with the community and stakeholders involved. He or she may be also be viewed as an outsider and lack the trust of community members. This disadvantage can be overcome by having respected community members on the leadership team who are visibly engaged in the process and supportive of the facilitator.

If an external facilitator is involved, it's important to remember that they are there to guide the process, not to develop a vision and plan for the community. Community leaders and members must be willing to put in the work and assume ownership (Center for Rural Pennsylvania, 2006; French & Gagne, 2010). This ensures that the resulting document is used to move the community forward toward its vision and doesn't just sit on a shelf or website.

Public and Key Stakeholder Engagement

To be effective and promote ownership, the community strategic visioning and planning process should include and engage people who reflect the political, racial, geographic, ethnic, and economic diversity of the community's residents, businesses, elected officials, local institutions, and other stakeholders (Center for Rural Pennsylvania, 2006; Okubo, 2000). This representation should occur at all levels and parts of the visioning and planning process—from members on the leadership team, subcommittees, and action committees to activities designed to solicit public and stakeholder input and mobilize people to action.

Community ownership can be characterized in terms of *process* (who has a voice and who is heard), *outcome* (who has influence over decisions and what happens as a result), and *distribution* (who is affected by the process and outcome) (Lachapelle, 2008). This is particularly important during the visioning stage. If a member of the community is unaware of the planning process, doesn't feel valued during the process or resulting decisions, or doesn't see his or her future in that vision, he or she is not likely to support the effort and may even work against it. Using a variety of methods gives more people a chance to participate in ways in which they feel comfortable and which fit into their schedules.

Community Surveys

When administered effectively, community surveys provide an opportunity to get input from a large audience to a standardized set of questions. In many communities, the same or similar surveys are conducted annually to inform planning activities as well as generate data with which to evaluate progress toward previously developed goals and objectives (Okubo, 2000). To provide quality data, care must be taken in designing survey questions and determining how the survey will be distributed to ensure you get the information you need to make appropriate decisions (Fowler, 2013; Okubo, 2000). Often different surveys are used to target different stakeholder groups, such as residents, youth, or business owners to solicit input on topics most relevant to them.

There are four primary ways of conducting self-administered surveys: group administration (distributed and collected in a group setting), drop-off (surveys that are dropped off to participants and mailed back or picked up), mail, and online (Fowler, 2013). To address limitations and maximize participation, consider using multiple distribution strategies.

- **Online surveys** have grown in popularity because they provide a low-cost and unintrusive way of collecting and analyzing data. The biggest downside is the potential for lack of participation among certain segments of the population who may lack internet access or digital literacy or simply choose not to respond.

- **Drop-off and mail surveys** often result in higher response rates than online surveys. However, they will cost more and require more effort than online surveys because they need to be printed, distributed, and collected. In addition, someone will have to tabulate results.

- **Group administration surveys** are relatively low in cost and typically have high response rates. However, the audience is limited to people at events where they are distributed. Also, people may be less thoughtful in responding to questions due to perceived time constraints. Like drop-off and mail surveys, group administration surveys will require the additional step of data entry and tabulation.

Regardless of form, when designing a community survey to solicit strong participation, a good rule of thumb is to make sure it can be completed in no more than 10 to 15 minutes. For comprehensive strategic plans, questions often cover a range of topics such as quality of life, community amenities, available services, local governance, business climate, and economic opportunities. Respondent demographics and background information are also gathered to identify populations that may need additional targeting to ensure adequate representation. You may also include a mix of open-ended questions as well as questions that ask those surveyed to rank or rate different aspects of the community or desired priorities.

Community Events

Community events can be an effective means of building ownership of the process, gathering data to inform efforts, and growing momentum for action and implementation. This can take a variety of forms.

Focus groups involve a small group of individuals who participate in a facilitated discussion about a specific topic where they can express their views in detail and hear the opinions of others (Lachapelle & Mastel, 2019). They can also be used to discuss technical and anecdotal information and engage participants in collective and creative problem solving. Since focus groups are based on open communication and critical deliberation, they can lead to improved community relations, trust, and a sense of ownership in the process and outcome. Focus groups are time-consuming and require a skilled facilitator to ensure engagement from all participants and keep the conversation focused on the topic at hand (Okubo, 2000). Focus groups are often used to gather more detailed information about a specific issue of interest that may have been identified through community surveys or at other points in the planning process. They may also be used to engage different stakeholder groups or segments of the population that are hard to reach through surveys or other engagement activities.

Public meetings are large gatherings where community members can learn about the strategic planning process, provide feedback, and volunteer to get involved (Okubo, 2000). They typically include a mix of presentations to share information with participants and facilitated exercises to engage them. Often these will be held at multiple points in the process, such as:

- a community kickoff event with visioning activities
- community dialogue sessions to conduct asset mapping and SWOT (Strengths, Weaknesses, Opportunities, Threats) analyses
- community input session to review proposed vision, goals, objectives, and strategies
- celebration event to unveil the final plan and kickoff implementation

A **charrette** is a series of meetings where community members and designers collaborate on a place-based vision for the community (Lennertz, Lutzenhise & Failor, 2008). Charrettes typically begin with a public workshop where participants work in small groups to describe and draw their vision. Groups present their top ideas to the other groups to develop common themes. A design team takes this information, meets with key stakeholders, and creates drawings or other visual depictions for members of the public to review and respond to. This process may be repeated until the design team reaches a final plan for the community. At this point, the effort transitions to an action planning process.

Action planning workshops typically occur in smaller group sessions where operational details are added to the strategic plan. Participants in these sessions will flesh out the who, what, when, where, and how related to different activities that will be performed to implement plan objectives and strategies. Action planning workshops may be conducted as part of the overall visioning and planning process with details included in the final plan, or they may be conducted after formal adoption of the plan as part of implementation. In either case, stakeholders and community members who have strong interest and want to be involved in implementation of the plan should be included in these sessions. This is important because communities don't implement plans, people do.

Communication

In order to foster buy-in and inclusiveness, communicating with the public throughout the process—to inform community members of progress and ways to get involved—should be intentional. Even in the smallest of communities, people look for and receive information in different ways, so it is important to use a variety of communications strategies (Okubo, 2000). While posting information on a website or social media accounts is a low-cost communication strategy, these efforts are not enough by themselves. Neither are news releases. Think through the political, racial, geographic, ethnic, and economic diversity of your community, then identity key partners who are connected to different segments of the population. Collaborate with those partners to determine how best to reach those different constituencies to keep them informed and encourage engagement. This could involve such channels as special events, organizational newsletters, employer bulletin boards, or fliers distributed at local businesses or churches. Then build and implement communications using those methods. In most instances, while time-consuming, nothing is as effective as a face-to-face or phone invitation from someone an individual trusts and respects.

Data to Inform Efforts

Data is important to ensuring that a community visioning and planning process is strategic and leads to desired results. Anyone can come up with a vision and plan for what they want. Ensuring that the vision and plan are a good fit for the community, however, often depends on the quality of the underlying data. Public engagement activities will provide a lot of data from the perspective of community members. However, the use of primary and secondary data providing an evidence-based picture of conditions and trends will ensure your plan is relevant and strategic (Miner & McDermand, 2003; Okubo, 2000; Taylor, 2019).

Examples of data often used in the visioning and planning process include:

- **Demographic:** population size, density, age, gender, racial and ethnic diversity, and migration patterns, as well as trends and projections of these characteristics over time

- **Economic:** wage and employment trends overall and by industry sector, business establishments, household income levels and sources, and poverty rates

- **Social:** health indicators, educational attainment, crime rates, insurance access

- **Community services and infrastructure:** availability and condition of utilities, broadband, roads and bridges, transportation, housing, education system, and access to healthcare

- **Quality of place:** cultural amenities, recreation and leisure opportunities, and social networks

Beyond analyzing data for your own community, it can be helpful to examine how your community compares to state, regional, national, or even global trends since these may reflect external forces that could impact you in the future (Okubo, 2000). It can also be helpful to compare your data to that of benchmark communities that are similar to yours or reflect your vision for the future.

In addition to informing the visioning and planning process, these data also provide a baseline from which to measure progress and success. For more information, see the chapter "Measuring Community Progress" in this handbook.

Detailed and Linked Priorities, Goals, and Action Plans

Once a vision for the future has been established, it's time to set priorities and begin fleshing out the details of the plan (Center for Rural Pennsylvania, 2006; Miner & McDermand, 2003). This process should utilize information gathered concerning the community's assets and strengths, trends and barriers affecting it, and opportunities for the future (Miner & McDermand, 2003; Okubo, 2000). The words used to describe different elements of the plan often vary, but the basic concepts are typically the same:

- **Priorities/goals/action areas:** These are the major themes or categories for which work will occur. They should directly or indirectly support the community's vision.

- **Strategies/objectives:** These are the major activities that will be carried out in support of each priority/goal/action area. During the planning process, community members may consider a variety of options but will ultimately need to prioritize which ones they can and should pursue. Factors influencing these decisions could include perceived importance, available resources, ease of accomplishment, and who is able and willing to do the work.

- **Action plan:** To facilitate implementation, an action plan defines in detail who, what, when, where and how each different strategy/objective will be achieved. While this information is often omitted from the formal published strategic plan, it is critical to facilitating implementation. It identifies the deliverables associated with the strategy/objective, the people responsible for carrying out specific tasks, and the time frames and deadlines for completing different activities. Having these details in place helps ensure ownership and accountability among community members. Exhibit C provides an example of these elements and how they relate to each other.

Two common problems with strategic plans—lack of clarity and attempts to tackle too much—may lead to failure in implementation. Goals explicitly linked to detailed strategies, objectives, and action steps should be clearly written so community members know what should be happening and what the intended results are. In addition, people involved in the strategic planning process need to be realistic about what is achievable with the manpower, time, and other resources available—and prioritize accordingly (Miner & McDermand, 2003). Start with those goals most important to community members and build from there in subsequent years. In most cases, it is better to successfully complete a few key strategies than to partially complete a large number of less important ones. That said, it can also be helpful to include actions that can create some quick early wins as well as others strategically accomplished at different points over time. The resulting energy helps community members feel that progress is being made and builds and sustains momentum moving forward.

Exhibit C. Example of Linkages between Priorities, Goals, and Action Plans

Vision: Townsville is a thriving community that actively engages its residents in improving quality of life and providing economic opportunities for all while respecting, preserving, and enhancing our community's natural resources and sense of place.

Priorities and Goals

Lifelong Learning	Investment in our Community	Investment in our Economy	Commitment toward our Future
We will provide quality formal and nonformal education that enables all residents to reach their career goals and sustains their families, and is responsive to needs of businesses and industry.	We will develop safe and affordable neighborhoods for all residents, quality healthcare, infrastructure for the future economy, and plentiful recreational and cultural opportunities.	We will listen to and be responsive to the needs of entrepreneurs, workers, and industry leaders to create a business environment that breeds success.	We will create an ecosystem of engagement where residents know their voices are heard and are able to play an active role in reaching our shared vision.

Strategies:[1]

Lifelong Learning Priority

- *Establish Education and Local Economy Task Force with representatives from local businesses and industry, the pre-K–12 educational system, and regional higher education to assess and regularly review workforce needs and training opportunities and determine whether current education programs are meeting those needs.*

- Create and expand job fairs, career expos, internships, and mentoring programs for youth and adults of all ages.

- Expand equitable offerings of high-quality early development programs, learning experiences, and related school readiness supports to position all children for success.

- Expand and enhance digital and technology skills of learners of all ages.

---

[1] Strategies for only one priority shown for illustrative purposes.

Action Plan:[2]

Priority—Lifelong Learning
Strategy –1. Education and Local Economy Task Force

Action Step	Lead Person	Individuals Involved	Target Completion Date	Date Completed	Notes
Hold meeting to develop proposal for task force structure and guidelines (representation, appointment process and terms, leadership structure, member responsibilities)	Mayor Susan	Strategic planning Lifelong Learning team	3/31/21	3/21/21	Mtg on 2/15/21; participants solicited feedback from missing stakeholders; completed draft at mtg on 3/18/21
Solicit stakeholder and public feedback on task force proposal	Mayor Susan	Mayor's office personnel	4/15/21		
Review proposal feedback and finalize task force structure and guidelines	Mayor Susan	Strategic planning Lifelong Learning team	6/30/21		
Appointment of task force members		TBD based on approved proposal	7/31/21		
First task force meeting			8/31/21		
And so on…					

[2] Actions for only one strategy shown for illustrative purposes.

Evaluation

Evaluation is an important and ongoing part of strategic visioning and planning. Communities engage in strategic visioning and planning because they want to achieve something—whether it be addressing social issues, ensuring continued quality of life and economic prosperity, or something else. A quality strategic plan will include strategies and action plans for measuring progress, including clearly defined metrics and indicators to gauge success in reaching the community's goals and vision (French & Gage, 2010; Miner & McDermand, 2003; Okubo, 2000). It will also embed activities to assess what is working with implementation—and what is not—and provide evidence to indicate when changes in direction are needed.

Tracking progress at the action plan level is typically straightforward and measured in terms of *process* (how the strategy is being implemented) and *outputs* (things we did). The purpose of this level of assessment is to answer the question, "Did we complete the things on our list to implement a particular strategy?" Identifying people with specific responsibilities and posting action plan progress on a chart—such as the one shown in Exhibit C—can help encourage follow-through during implementation.

At the strategy level, evaluation of progress may involve a combination of tracking outputs and *outcomes* (what happened because of what we did). Outcomes usually take longer to achieve and require tracking indicators over time. They may also be impacted by factors beyond the community's control.

Using the highlighted example in Exhibit C (*Lifelong Learning Priority, Strategy 1*), examples of output measures might include:

- number of times the Education and Local Economy Task Force met
- number of businesses surveyed
- number of educational programs reviewed and/or changed

Outcome measure examples might include:
- reduced unemployment rates for local K–12 and higher education graduates
- higher household incomes
- reduction in business expenses to provide remedial training for new hires
- reduced in-migration of workers from outside the community.

As part of the planning process, community members must decide what success looks like for each strategy and what indicators will be used to measure and track it. As discussed in previous sections, these data might come from primary data sources such as surveys or secondary sources. For more information, see the chapter "Measuring Community Progress" in this handbook.

If the actions and strategies being implemented are not leading to desired outcomes, the community will need to investigate why. It could be a problem with process, such as a lack of follow-through, the inability to engage people who need to be involved to complete a task or strategy, or a lack of other necessary resources. Alternatively, it could be that the community is measuring the wrong thing or that the strategies being pursued are the wrong ones for achieving desired outcomes. In this situation, community leaders may want to contact their regional or state economic development agency or other community and economic development organizations for assistance.

Strategic visioning and planning is not a one-and-done process (Miner & McDermand, 2003). Planned and regular evaluation is needed to pivot and make changes when things aren't working. It also allows local leaders to adjust or change course in response to external forces and trends that impact the community or changes within the community itself.

Celebration

While often overlooked, celebration is an important part of the visioning, planning, and implementation process (Nagy & Fawcett, 2006; Okubo, 2000). Activities and events that recognize contributions of community members, showcase accomplishments, and simply allow people to socialize and have fun together are important to create an environment in which people want to be involved. Hosting events such as community potlucks or picnics helps prevent volunteer burnout, remind people of their shared visions and aspirations, and draw new people into community efforts moving forward. Activities that reflect and celebrate your community's unique character will likely be the most meaningful. Sprinkling these frequently through the year make the process a positive experience for those involved and encourages continued involvement. Capturing these memories and publicizing them through the media, social media, and community records will extend that positivity beyond the events themselves.

Case Study
Cleveland County, Arkansas

Cleveland County, Arkansas (population 8,689) is slowly overcoming 21 years of limited economic development, change, and improvements. Faced with vacant storefronts, declining population, and a stagnant economy, community leaders in the city of Rison came together in 2012 to discuss how to take action. This led to formation of Rison Shine Downtown Development, a grassroots organization dedicated to revitalizing downtown Rison. Rison Shine created the first Cleveland County Christmas Parade, a pocket park, and a new farmers' market.

After discussion with the local leaders, the group decided to expand their efforts county-wide. These visionary leaders recognized that:

- It is important to work together as a county because what impacts one part of the county impacts the whole county.

- Together we can do things we could never do by ourselves, because we will have more resources and assets to work with.

- Together we can shape our county's future for our children and grandchildren.

In February 2015, leaders from Cleveland County partnered with the University of Arkansas System Division of Agriculture Cooperative Extension Service to begin a strategic community visioning and planning process as part of Extension's Breakthrough Solutions program. This led to the launch of Kick Start Cleveland County, a county-wide grassroots effort to create economic opportunities and improve the quality of life for all of Cleveland County.

The visioning and planning process followed four basic steps: (1) Discover—Trends, Assets and Key Drivers; (2) Dream—Describe Your Desired Future; (3) Design—Identify Key Priorities; and (4) Deliver—Strategies and Action Plans.

After organizational meetings with the core leadership team in late spring, a county-wide Asset Opportunity Tour was held in June 2015. Also that month, Cleveland County was one of two counties featured in the Breakthrough Solutions Pre-Conference Branding Workshop, which led to creation of the county's brand (*America's Homestead—Real. Simple. Life*), building off two key assets in the county, the Pioneer Village and a highly successful homesteading conference held in Rison that has served as a catalyst for homesteading conferences across the state and region. A community survey was also conducted that summer.

With strong community involvement, four working sessions were held throughout the summer and fall to:

- develop the county's vision statement for the next five to ten years;

- identify core values;

- form action teams to work on key priorities; and

- establish an organizational structure to establish roles for moving forward and sustaining the initiative once the county transitioned to implementation.

A hub-and-spoke structure was chosen, with the hub (the large group) making overarching decisions regarding process, and action teams tackling issues, pursuing opportunities, and engaging stakeholders related to their individual priorities. The Kick Start Cleveland County Blueprint and Action Plan was officially approved and launched in November 2015.

Continued commitment to the cause, investment and leveraging of assets, and making the most of opportunities that fit with the vision and goals developed by the citizens of Cleveland County have resulted in significant breakthroughs and are making a sustained difference. Action teams have continued their work since 2015. Each year, they host a Kick Start Cleveland County Celebration to keep community members aware of ongoing efforts, recognize a "Volunteer of the Year" from each action team, and celebrate their accomplishments. Major accomplishments in 2020 included collaborative agreements to build the new Kingsland Heritage Center, which will focus on the birthplace and ancestral home of Johnny Cash; six shows by the Cleveland County Community Theater reaching more than 900 attendees with $11,540 in ticket sales; 36 community events reaching 15,214 people; and $79,840 generated through donations, grants, and in-kind program support to support the efforts of action teams.

References

Center for Rural Pennsylvania. (2006). *Planning for the future: A handbook on community visioning* (3rd ed.). https://www.rural.palegislature.us/visioning3.pdf.

Fowler, F. (2013). *Survey research methods* (5th ed.). Sage Publications.

French, C.A. & Gagne, M. (2010). Ten years of community visioning in New Hampshire: the meaning of "success." *Journal of the Community Development Society, 41*(2), 223–239.

Hinz, L. (n.d). *Pros and cons of using internal and external facilitators.* University of Minnesota Extension. https://extension.umn.edu/public-engagement-strategies/pros-and-cons-using-internal-and-external-facilitators.

Lachapelle, P. (2008). A sense of ownership in community development: understanding the potential for participation in community planning efforts. *Journal of the Community Development Society,* 39(2), 52–59.

Lachapelle, P., Emery, M. & Hays, R.L. (2010). The pedagogy and the practice of community visioning: Evaluating effective community strategic planning in rural Montana. *Journal of the Community Development Society,* 41(2), 176–191.

Lachapelle, P. & Mastel, T. (2019). Using focus groups for community development. *Community Planning and Zoning.* https://community-planning.extension.org/using-focus-groups-for-community-development.

Lennertz, B., Lutzenhiser, A. & Failor, T. (2008). An introduction to charrettes. *Planning Commissioners Journal, 71.* http://plannersweb.com/wp-content/uploads/2012/07/262.pdf.

Miner, P. & McDermand, D. (2003). *Developing a community strategic plan: A guide for local officials.* Illinois Association of Regional Councils in partnership with Department of Commerce and Economic Opportunity. https://ilarconline.org/file/8/StrategicPlanGuide.pdf.

Nagy, J. & Fawcett, S.B. (n.d). An overview of strategic planning or "VMOSA" (Vision, Mission, Objectives, Strategies, and Action Plans). In *Community Tool Box*. Center for Community Health and Development, University of Kansas. https://ctb.ku.edu/en/table-of-contents/structure/strategic-planning/vmosa/main.

Okubo, D. (2000). *The community visioning and strategic planning handbook.* National Civic League Press. http://mrsc.org/getmedia/D9ADE917-2DF1-4EA2-9AA8-14D713F5CE98/VSPHandbook.aspx.

Taylor, G. (2019). Elements of a comprehensive plan. *Community Planning and Zoning.* https://community-planning.extension.org/elements-of-a-comprehensive-plan.

Identifying and Developing Stakeholders, Leaders, and Volunteers

Lesley Graybeal, PhD

This chapter focuses on processes and strategies used to identify and develop stakeholders and volunteers. Strategically utilizing and aligning these two groups to achieve community goals is important to the success of our communities. Each group brings something unique to the table.

Learning Outcomes

- Participants will review the basics of stakeholder engagement, leadership development, and volunteer recruitment, recognition, and retention.

- Participants will understand strategies for utilizing stakeholders and leaders and managing volunteers for maximum effectiveness.

- Participants will discuss the pros and cons of using volunteers in a variety of situations.

- Participants will learn the value of team building and cooperation in communities.

Volunteering is defined as activities performed in formal settings in which time is freely given to benefit others without remuneration (Cnaan, Handy & Wadsworth, 1996). According to AmeriCorps (n.d.), 77.4 million Americans volunteered in 2019 for a total of 6.9 billion hours, contributing a value of $167 billion to nonprofit and government organizations and communities. The organizations that these volunteers served were most often religious organizations (32%), organizations devoted to arts and culture, sports or a particular hobby (26%), or educational or youth service organizations (19%), and the most common activities performed by volunteers in

2019 included fundraising; collecting, preparing, or serving food; collecting, making, or distributing clothing or other goods; mentoring; and tutoring or teaching.

Yet volunteer engagement is not only significant for its economic impact as a form of labor or for the services that it provides in communities; volunteer engagement is also an important source of social capital for communities across the United States. Volunteers become stakeholders in the organizations and communities that they serve and can develop strong ties to one another, to organizational leaders, and to fellow community members served. This social capital benefits not only the volunteers and the organizations themselves, but communities as a whole.

Stakeholder Engagement

From high school or college students interested in discovering their own interests and developing professional skills, to professionals seeking opportunities to build their networks or reinforce bonds within teams, to older adults hoping to stay engaged and contribute to a cause that they care about, our communities are full of diverse stakeholders with unique motivations for giving their time and talents to the places they call home. When it comes to engaging and managing stakeholders and volunteers, the theories and concepts most often brought to bear come from the field of human resource management, since volunteers often interact with organizations in a parallel manner to paid staff. Yet human resource management cannot perfectly account for all of the necessary dimensions of engaging community stakeholders as volunteers. Therefore, before considering a comprehensive management strategy for volunteers, organization and community leaders must first understand the types of roles and opportunities for volunteers as well as some of the common models an organization's volunteer management strategies may follow.

Models for Volunteer Involvement

Research on volunteer management has demonstrated the importance of an approach that aligns volunteer roles to the mission, organizational structure, and capacity of the organization rather than implementing a one-size-fits-all strategy. Some patterns emerge across organizations and opportunities, however, and one way of categorizing volunteer roles is presented by Sarah Jane Rehnborg in *Strategic Volunteer Engagement: A Guide for Nonprofit and Public Sector Leaders* (2009). Rehnborg's volunteer involvement framework represents types of volunteer roles in a matrix, with each role taking place along two continuums: time and connection. Roles may require a short-term, episodic commitment or a longer-term, ongoing commitment; additionally, volunteers may be primarily connected to the service through the skill that they contribute to the role or, for less skilled positions, through the affiliation that they have with the organization, its mission, or the population it serves. Table 1 presents four examples of volunteer roles, one in each quadrant of the matrix.

Table 1

Examples of volunteer roles by time and connection to service

	Connection to Service	
Time for Service	*Affiliation Focus*	*Skill Focus*
Episodic	A team of corporate volunteers participating in a one-day clean-up project	A service-learning class creating deliverables such as brochues or videos
Ongoing	A retiree or parent serving as a Sunday School teacher or scout troop leader	A young professional serving on a nonprofit board to offer expertise

Adapted from Rehnborg (2009)

In addition to understanding how different types of volunteer involvement demand different time commitments and skill levels, volunteer managers can benefit from understanding how different organizations may adopt different models for their interactions with volunteers more broadly. In Table 2, Jeffrey Brudney and Lucas C.P.M. Meijs (2014) represent how four models of involving volunteers require different types of relationships between the organization and the volunteer—including the role of the volunteer, recruitment of the volunteer, volunteer motivation, volunteer management, and relationship of volunteer to organizational governance. The four models of volunteer involvement (adapted from Rochester, 1999) are service delivery, support role, member/activist, and coworker.

Table 2

Four models of volunteer involvement

Relationship to Volunteer	Type of Model			
	Service Delivery Model	Support Role Model	Member/Activist Model	Co-worker Model
Role of volunteer	Most of work done by volunteer	Volunteer supplement work of paid staff	All positions held by volunteers	Unclear distinctions between volunteer and paid staff
Recruitment of volunteer	Specific recruitment based on volunteer availability	Volunteer recruited to take a non-operational role	Volunteer's purpose in organization is self-defined	Volunteer's purpose in organization is self-defined
Volunteer management	"Workplace model"	Part "workplace," part teamwork	Teamwork, personal leadership	Teamwork, personal leadership
Relationship of volunteer to governance	Clear differentiation between volunteer and paid staff	Somewhwat clear differentiation between volunteer and paid staff	No paid staff, organization governed by member activists	Ambiguous difference between volunteer and paid staff

From "Models of Volunteer Management: Professional Volunteer Program Management in Social Work," by Jeffrey L. Brudney & Lucas C.P.M. Meijs, 2014, p. 12. Adapted from Rochester, 1999.

As Brudney and Meijs' analysis shows, volunteers who are involved in service delivery often have roles that resemble or even replicate paid staff roles and thus have a hierarchical relationship with organizational staff; by contrast, volunteers with organizations that are focused on mutual aid or advocacy often have more voice or a greater management role by virtue of the fact that the organization is itself volunteer-led. Just as each volunteer may be able to make different time commitments, may have different skills to contribute, or may have a different affiliation with the organization they serve, each of the four models presented in Table 2 may appeal to different volunteers depending on their motivations or their management preferences.

Volunteer Management

Just as management practices can be instrumental in the success or failure of for-profit organizations, the management of volunteers in nonprofit or government organizations can lead to successful outcomes for the organization and the community overall, or to failure to engage or retain stakeholders in the community. A volunteer management plan that aligns volunteer roles with larger organizational and community goals, while also supporting those volunteer roles (Rogers, Rogers & Boyd, 2013), can prevent many of the common challenges that the people (often volunteers themselves) tasked with coordinating volunteers face. Rather than following a linear process, volunteer management constitutes a cycle beginning with the establishment of volunteer roles, continuing to the recruitment and development of volunteers, and concluding with the recognition and retention (or separation) of volunteers (Figure 1).

Figure 1

The volunteer management process

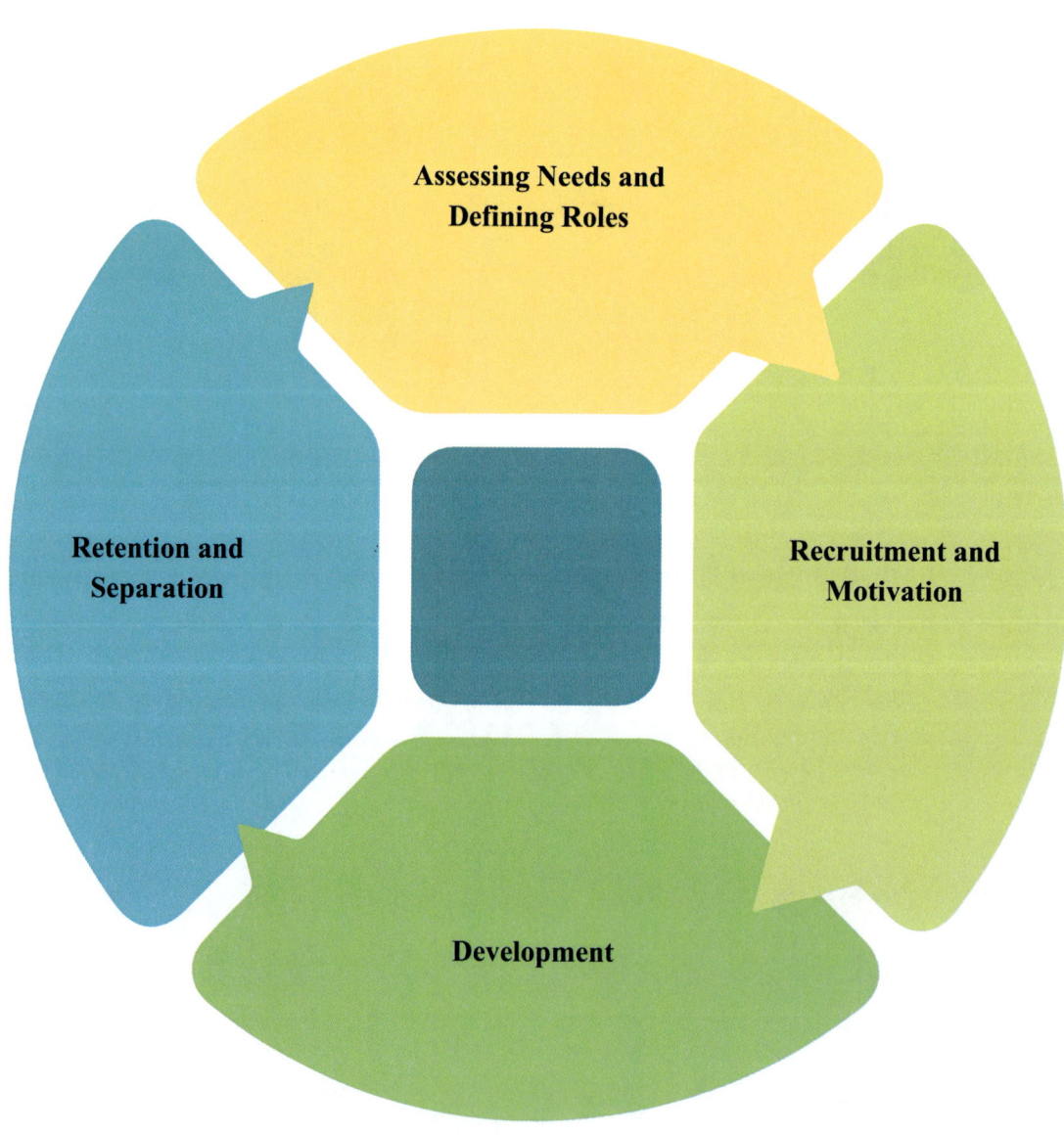

Assessing Needs and Defining Roles

The initial stage of a volunteer management plan should include an assessment of the organization's structure, size, budget, capacity to manage volunteers, services, and overall mission and goals. An organization that has limited staff availability to manage volunteers may need to reassign responsibilities or resources in order to establish a successful volunteer program, while an organization going through a difficult financial time may not find a volunteer program to be worth the investment required for recruiting, training, and recognizing volunteers. Without a shared understanding of the organization and what it hopes to accomplish a volunteer program, organizational leaders and volunteer managers will struggle to define successful roles for volunteers to fill.

The second essential part of the initial stage of volunteer management planning is to define the roles of volunteers. As Brudney and Meijs (2014) established, volunteers may be used to provide a specific set of services within the organization (e.g., at a homeless shelter that allows volunteers to prepare and serve meals), may supplement or assist with the work of paid staff (e.g,. at a camp where volunteers serve as assistant counselors), or may in fact manage the organization or be indistinguishable from paid staff (e.g,. in a policy organization with a large group of volunteer advocates or lobbyists). Regardless of what role a volunteer will fulfill, organizations should have a position description outlining the scope of the volunteer's duties and responsibilities, expectations, time commitment, and other key information to help volunteers navigate their relationships with their supervisor and the organization.

Recruitment and Motivation

Once an organization has established the need for and roles of volunteers, a volunteer coordinator can begin recruiting community members to fill volunteer roles. Effective volunteer recruitment stems from an understanding of the motivations that drive volunteers to get involved and requires effective communication of organizational values and expectations. Functional motives theory (Clary & Snyder, 1999) describes six functions that volunteering fulfills for the individual:

- **Values Motive:** Volunteering affirms and allows people to express their values by contributing to causes that they care about.

- **Understanding Motive:** Volunteering provides people with new experiences and opportunities to learn and grow.

- **Social Motive:** Volunteering allows people to make or reinforce social connections, or have their efforts affirmed by others.

- **Career Motive:** Volunteering enhances people's employability, both through professional skills development and resume building.

- **Protective Motive:** Volunteering combats negative feelings by giving people opportunities to minimize their own problems or alleviate guilt over their good fortune.
- **Enhancement Motive:** Volunteering increases positive feelings by increasing people's self-esteem, confidence, and efficacy.

Recruitment strategies should speak to one of more of these motivations, and volunteer managers should seek to understand the motivations that are most salient for their organization's volunteers in particular in order to reinforce and reward them throughout the volunteer experience.

In addition to understanding the factors that motivate volunteers to get involved, volunteer managers must be able to effectively communicate how available volunteer opportunities align with these motivations. Recruitment tools such as organization websites, press releases announcing the launch of a new volunteer program, social media accounts, and position listings in online volunteer databases must all clearly articulate the organization's mission and values, as well as accurately portray what volunteers will learn and do as part of the organization.

Development

Sometimes termed the *performance assurance* stage of volunteer management (Studer & von Schnurbein, 2013), development of volunteers is crucial to the success of the projects to which volunteers contribute. Development of volunteers may include initial training and orientation, as well as ongoing professional development opportunities and strategies for including volunteers as valued members of the team. Development of volunteers may also involve preventing or resolving conflicts, which is often accomplished through liability waivers, confidentiality agreements, photo or video release forms, safety policies, professionalism standards, and other policies and procedures covered in a volunteer handbook and a signed volunteer agreement.

Organization leaders often have performance management systems in place for paid staff members but should find ways to include volunteers in existing systems or develop parallel systems for evaluating volunteers' work. While organizations can easily measure the number of volunteers involved and hours completed, other ways of assessing impact can include funds or donations raised, client satisfaction, or progress towards mutually agreed-upon goals. Measuring the contributions of volunteers can not only help volunteers to see the impact of their work and feel a sense of accomplishment, but performance can also be used to determine volunteer rewards and recognition.

From onboarding to more advanced

training or evolution of roles, development of volunteers can significantly increase volunteers' confidence in their ability to perform their roles (Newton, Becker & Bell, 2014), their motivation to serve an organization that shares their values (Zievinger & Swint, 2018), and their commitment to continue to volunteer.

Retention and Separation

Retention of qualified volunteers is frequently reported by nonprofit leaders as the greatest challenge of volunteer management (Hurst, Scherer & Allen, 2017). In addition to volunteer training, the support and recognition that volunteers receive during and after their service also contribute to volunteer motivation and, in turn, volunteer retention. Nonprofit research has revealed, perhaps unsurprisingly, that the more motivated volunteers are, the longer they stay with the organizations they serve (Zievinger & Swint, 2018).

Supporting Volunteers

A common mistake of volunteer managers is to assume that volunteer attrition is largely due to factors that are personal or intrinsic to the volunteer. In fact, volunteers who feel supported by the organization, who feel that they have a voice in the organization's operations, and who feel that their work with the organization matters are more likely to persist in their volunteer positions over time (Hurst, Scherer & Allen, 2017; Mayr, 2017). In order to ensure that volunteers feel supported in their roles, volunteer managers should always make intended outcomes for volunteers clear in the recruitment and development stages.

Organizations can also develop systems of peer support for volunteers through a volunteer corps or cohort structure. Such a system of support can allow for simpler delivery of ongoing training for volunteers, reinforce the social motivation for volunteering, and increase volunteers' affinity to the group and likelihood of staying involved. Effective volunteer managers will ensure that volunteers feel connected to one another, to the organization, and to the impact of the organization on the community.

Rewarding Volunteers

Volunteers may feel intrinsically rewarded by relationships developed with other stakeholders, by meaningful or creative work as a member of the organization, or by the impact that they have on the community. Organizations can also reward volunteers through advancement by structuring volunteer roles to allow experienced volunteers to take on greater responsibility over time or with additional training. Such a structure for volunteer advancement additionally reinforces volunteers' motivations related to understanding and career development.

Organizations can also provide a variety of extrinsic types of rewards to recognize their volunteers and maintain their involvement. Organizations should make an effort to recognize volunteers in a general way—such as thanking all the volunteers at an event or providing perks such as snacks or t-shirts—as well as on an individual basis at key milestones in their volunteer careers. Some studies of volunteer recognition programs have shown that volunteer awards can serve as valuable incentives, making those who receive them feel recognized and leading others to aspire to receive them in the future (Frey & Gallus, 2018). Awards can be either *confirmatory* or *discretionary*, with confirmatory awards given out to all volunteers who meet certain criteria (such as a defined number of volunteer hours or length of volunteer service) and discretionary awards recognizing exceptional volunteers.

Volunteer Separation

Of course, very few volunteers will continue to serve the same organization indefinitely, so separation is also part of the volunteer management process. Whether organizations need to release a volunteer from service due to poor performance or say goodbye to an exceptional volunteer stepping back from long-held responsibilities, the separation stage can be an opportunity for volunteer managers to seek feedback on their own processes and even solicit leads for new volunteers. Organizations should never miss the opportunity to learn from their outgoing volunteers, using tools such as volunteer satisfaction surveys after an episodic event or experience and exit interviews for long-term volunteers. Feedback received from volunteers can inform organization leaders in reassessing the need for volunteers and revising volunteer roles, training, and rewards, completing the cycle of volunteer management.

The Reciprocal Relationship between Volunteers and Organizations

Rebecca Nesbit and colleagues (2017) have grouped dimensions of volunteer involvement into two categories: organization choices and volunteer choices. Organizations choose whether and how to use volunteers, how many volunteers to engage, and what the status of volunteers will be in the organization overall. Volunteers simultaneously make choices about when to start and end their involvement with an organization, how deeply to get involved, and how much to contribute. Neither the organization nor the volunteer can make these choices without the other, making their relationship a reciprocal one. The choices that organizations make about how to engage volunteers affect the choices that volunteers make about how to engage with the organization and vice versa. Volunteers are true stakeholders in the nonprofit and government organizations that they serve, and volunteer programs thus act as feedback loops that both reflect and drive changes in the community. Organizational leaders and volunteer managers must be aware of how changes that they make to their volunteer programs may impact their ability to recruit and retain volunteers, and they must also be attentive to how changes to their volunteer pool may create new possibilities for volunteer roles or recruitment strategies.

Inclusion and Innovation in Volunteer Management

A strong volunteer management strategy will plan not only for the volunteers that an organization has had in the past but also for the volunteers of the future. Whether adapting to demographic changes in their local communities or the nation as a whole, or developing plans to engage specific types of volunteers, organizations must equip themselves to work with increasingly diverse populations of volunteers.

Engaging Diverse Populations of Volunteers

Organizations and communities that wish to increase their volunteer participation should be attentive to the changing demographics of the volunteer pool (Nesbit & Brudney, 2013). These changing demographics include a larger proportion of Latinx and African American volunteers, as well as volunteers over the age of 65. These demographic changes should also drive changes to volunteer recruitment messaging, volunteer roles, and volunteer rewards.

Recruitment of volunteers from racial and cultural groups outside of the volunteer manager's own requires relationship building. Volunteer managers can use targeted recruitment of individuals through religious and cultural institutions rather than general advertisement. Different groups of people have different motivations for volunteering and seek different types of volunteer activities and rewards from the experience, so recognizing and understanding these differences is a crucial skill of volunteer managers who wish to develop sustainable and adaptable volunteer programs. A very effective tool for building trust among a group of community members who have not previously been engaged with the organization is to increase representation among the organization's leadership and other paid staff. Research has shown that members of racial minority groups are more likely to volunteer for organizations that serve, employ, or are led by members of their racial group (Nesbit & Brudney, 2013). Organizations should strive to create robust diversity, equity, and inclusion policies in order to hire and retain paid staff and support recruitment of volunteers from diverse groups in the community as well.

Engaging College Student Volunteers

For organizations in communities that are also home to higher education institutions, college students can simultaneously be incredibly valuable to nonprofits and challenging for volunteer managers. College students often bring diverse backgrounds and perspectives to a community and to organizations where they volunteer, and they may also be in a position to apply newly acquired skills or knowledge in a volunteer setting. At the same time, studies of nonprofit engagement of college student volunteers have revealed that college students' schedule constraints, the many demands they balance, and their transience during breaks in the academic calendar typically do not fit organizations' needs (Jones, Giles & Carroll, 2019). Higher education institutions can help to address some of the challenges for organizations by coaching faculty and students in how to prepare for meaningful interactions with community organizations. Additionally, higher education institutions can provide an infrastructure for helping organizations recruit and retain college student volunteers, including a dedicated staff position responsible for developing and maintaining partnerships, an annual volunteer fair event, and recognition for students who make long-term rather than episodic service commitments.

Organizations that wish to tap into the talent, energy, and diverse perspectives of college students can develop recognition programs that emphasize longevity, support volunteers' professional development and career readiness, and create robust onboarding processes to ensure that only committed volunteers are recruited. Additionally, organizations may be able to adapt their volunteer roles to provide opportunities that align with the academic calendar and leverage existing volunteer involvement to create long-term relationships with student organizations or academic departments. Even as individual students come and go from the university, a long-term relationship with a specific campus organization or department can supply a nonprofit with a reliable source of episodic volunteers if the relationship is maintained.

Engaging Older Volunteers

Just as college students represent a unique pool of likely volunteers in communities that are home to higher education institutions, retired community members frequently seek opportunities to stay engaged in the community through volunteer service. Older volunteers also bring unique benefits and challenges to the organizations they work with. Retirees typically have a large body of knowledge, advanced skills, and professional expertise that can be put to use for organizations, whether they are helping to deliver services or acting as nonprofit board members. Additionally, retirees may belong to multiple other community organizations, including faith communities and civic clubs, and so may be effective advocates, fundraisers, and volunteer recruiters for the organizations that they serve. Older volunteers are frequently some of the most reliable and dedicated volunteers at an organization as well, and are often willing to make long-term commitments to serve.

At the same time, organizations must be attentive to the health and safety needs of all volunteers, making sure that physical spaces in which volunteers serve are accessible and that roles are available that can accommodate volunteers with a range of sensory or mobility needs. As with college students, organizations can capitalize on the many assets of older volunteers with volunteer management that is mindful and strategic.

Using Technology for Volunteer Management

Changes to volunteer demographics also often necessitate changes in how volunteer managers interact with volunteers. While some volunteers prefer to learn about volunteer opportunities from in-person interactions, technology provides a gateway for organizations to have unprecedented access to potential volunteers and stakeholders. Most organizations use technology to some degree to recruit and manage volunteers, such as keeping an electronic list of volunteers and their contact information, sending an email newsletter to past volunteers with upcoming opportunities, or sending text reminders to volunteers signed up for a service event.

A number of robust volunteer management tools are available to organizations that wish to streamline their procedures or expand their data collection and analysis capabilities. Volunteer websites such as VolunteerMatch and GivePulse allow organizations to create public profiles and event listings, register volunteers electronically, and track volunteer hours. Such tools not only allow organizations to more readily access younger volunteers, but they also can generate national visibility for an organization willing to offer remote or virtual service opportunities to volunteers from outside the local community.

Managing Volunteers in a Disaster

Volunteer managers face a unique set of challenges when dealing with the volunteers who show up in the wake of a disaster (also referred to as convergent volunteers) (Sigman, 2018). When a community's emergency management plan fails to account for *convergent volunteers*, these volunteers are underutilized or even unwelcome. Emergency management officials should plan for the reality that well-intentioned but untrained volunteers are likely to be present. Convergent volunteers may require training, protective equipment, and appropriate tools, and—most importantly—coordination. Identifying sites to serve as volunteer centers can provide screening, orientation, and placement for convergent volunteers while providing a buffer between a potentially overwhelming number of volunteers and changing on-the-ground needs.

Weighing the Benefits and Challenges of Volunteer Management

Volunteer retention and reliability present the greatest threat to organizations' volunteer programs and overall operations (Vantilborgh & Van Puyvelde, 2018). While volunteers may be deployed in vital roles, in comparison with paid employees, volunteers have fewer incentives to remain involved, have more fragmented commitments to the organization, and may be less bound by their affiliation to the organization. Given these differences, organizations have less power to enforce role expectations with volunteers.

Some organizations may decide that the costs of unreliable volunteers outweigh the potential benefits of a volunteer program. In fact, research has shown that the greater a nonprofit's reliance on earned income from commercial activities (such as sale of goods or services rendered), the less willing the organization is to engage volunteers (Lee, 2019). As organizations require more professionalized staff and greater cost consciousness, the investment that organizations must make in a volunteer program becomes harder to justify. Yet beyond the labor that they provide, volunteers also provide benefits—albeit less tangible or measurable benefits—by acting as liaisons between the organizations they serve and the community (Morris et al., 2017). Organizations that recognize and reinforce this role can increase their community visibility and efficiency in delivering services.

Regardless of the challenge that volunteer managers perceive, a strategic system for volunteer management can transform a challenge of volunteer engagement into an asset for the organization. Volunteer managers and community stakeholders alike will find themselves frustrated when the motivations, skills, and preferences of interested volunteers and the current volunteer management infrastructure are misaligned (Rogers, Rogers & Boyd, 2013). Rather than viewing changing volunteer demographics or unique populations of volunteers as a problem, however, skilled volunteer managers who embrace the reciprocal relationship between volunteers and nonprofit organizations can respond with innovative volunteer programs that effectively leverage available resources for the benefit of all.

Empowering Volunteers as for Grassroots Community Development

Effective volunteer management can look very different from one organization or community to the next, depending on the organization's size and capacity, leadership, mission and values, and the services that the organization provides. Nearly all sectors of our communities are able to engage volunteers with some careful planning, however, from local government, education, medical, and human services to the environment, community organizing and advocacy, and emergency management. Volunteers can be an invaluable resource for organizations and communities by sharing their time, skills, and commitments. Perhaps the greatest value of volunteer engagement, however, is the development of volunteers as stakeholders empowered to support one another and improve our communities.

Case Study
Creating Partnerships for Volunteer Engagement

The Faulkner County Juvenile Court in Conway, Arkansas, recognized the need for a robust volunteer management strategy when it implemented a new risk assessment tool to help identify the specific needs of the young people adjudicated by the court. Identifying the underlying causes of young people's behavior was of little use without programs and interventions that could help address the needs of youth and their families.

The court's chief of staff took on the responsibility of reaching out to community stakeholders, including civic organizations, nonprofits, and higher education institutions, to establish a range of new programs led by skilled volunteers willing to make a long-term commitment to court-involved youth. University students and professors led boxing clubs and tutoring sessions, while retirees offered sewing classes and young professionals taught fitness lessons. Each lead volunteer was responsible for recruiting and managing any additional volunteers needed for a program, while the chief of staff managed the necessary background checks, provided training to volunteers, and coordinated letters of recognition—signed by the judge—for each volunteer.

The court's use of strategic partnerships to mobilize a diverse range of community volunteers to offer a suite of new services for court-involved youth was highly successful in achieving desired outcomes. The local community saw drastically lower rates of juvenile crime and recidivism, and the court became a model for others in the state looking to achieve similar results. Connecting all the court's new programs, volunteers, and beneficiaries was the belief that court-involved youth belong to the community and that their own contributions as community members are irreplaceable.

References

AmeriCorps. (n.d.). Volunteering in America. https://www.nationalservice.gov/serve/via

Brudney, J.L. & Meijs, L.C.P.M. (2014). Models of volunteer management: Professional volunteer program management in social work. *Human Service Organizations: Management, Leadership, and Governance, 38*, 297–309. https://doi.org/10.1080/23303131.2014.899281

Clary, E.G.G. & Snyder, M. (1999). The motivations to volunteer: Theoretical and practical considerations. *Current Directions in Psychological Science, 8*(5), 156–159.

Cnaan, R.A., Handy, F. & Wadsworth, M. (1996). Defining who is a volunteer: Conceptual and empirical considerations. *Nonprofit and Voluntary Sector Quarterly, 25*(3), 364–383.

Frey, B.S. & Gallus, J. (2018). Volunteer organizations: Motivating with awards. In R. Ranyard (Ed.), *Economic psychology* (pp. 273–286). Wiley.

Hurst, C., Scherer, L. & Allen, J. (2017). Distributive justice for volunteers: Extrinsic outcomes matter. *Nonprofit Management and Leadership, 27*(3), 411–421. https://doi.org/10.1002/nml.21251

Jones, J.A., Giles, E. & Carroll, E. (2019). Student volunteers in a college town: Burden or lifeblood for the voluntary sector? *Journal of Service-Learning in Higher Education, 9.*

Lee, Y. (2019). Variations in volunteer use among human service organizations in the USA. *Voluntas, 30,* 208-221. https://doi.org/10.1007/s11266-018-9969-y

Mayr, M.L. (2017). Transformational leadership and volunteer firefighter engagement: The mediating role of group identification and perceived social impact. *Nonprofit Management and Leadership, 28*(2), 259–270. https://doi.org/10.1002/nml.21279

Morris, S.M., Payne, S., Ockenden, N. & Hill, M., (2017). Hospice volunteers: Bridging the gap to the community? *Health and Social Care in the Community, 25*(6), 1704–1713. https://doi.org/10.1111/hsc.12232

Nesbit, R. & Brudney, J.L. (2013). The implications of the Serve America Act for volunteer diversity and management. *Nonprofit Management and Leadership, 24*(1), 3–21.

Nesbit, R., Christensen, R.K. & Brudney, J.L. (2017). The limits and possibilities of volunteering: A framework for explaining the scope of volunteer involvement in public and nonprofit organizations. *Public Administration Review, 78*(4), 502–513.

Newton, C., Becker, K. & Bell, S. (2014). Learning and development opportunities as a tool for the retention of volunteers: A motivational perspective. *Human Resource Management Journal, 24*(4), 514–530. https://doi.org/10.1111/puar.12894

Rehnborg, S. J. (2009). *Strategic volunteer engagement: A guide for nonprofit and public sector leaders.* RGK Center for Philanthropy & Community Service, University of Texas at Austin. http://www.volunteeralive.org/docs/Strategic%20Volunteer%20Engagement.pdf

Rochester, C. (1999.) One size does not fit all: Four models of involving volunteers in voluntary organizations. *Voluntary Action, 1*(2), 47–59.

Rogers, S.E., Rogers, C.M., & Boyd, K.D. (2013). Challenges and opportunities in healthcare volunteer management: Insights from volunteer administrators. *Hospital Topics, 91*(2), 43–51. https://doi.org/10.1080/00185868.2013.806012

Sigman, R.K. (2018). Ethical dilemmas presented by convergent volunteers during emergency response. *Journal of Business Continuity & Emergency Planning, 12*(1), 56–62.

Studer, S. & von Schnurbein, G. (2013). Organization factors affecting volunteers: A literature review on volunteer coordination. *Voluntas, 24,* 403–440. https://doi.org/10.1007/s11266-012-9268-y

Vantilborgh, T. & Van Puyvelde, S. (2018). Volunteer reliability in nonprofit organizations: A theoretical model. *Voluntas, 29*, 29–42. https://doi.org/10.1007/s11266-017-9909-2

Zievinger, D. & Swint, F. (2018). Retention of festival volunteers: Management practices and volunteer motivation. *Research in Hospitality Management, 8*(2), 107–114. https://doi.org/10.1080/22243534.2018.1553374

Understanding Community Economies

Corey Parks, PCED & Jamie Gates, CCE

Understanding how local economies function and grow is an important subject for everyone involved in community and economic development to understand. Knowledge of this topic makes for more informed decisions regarding improving the standard of living and quality of life for all citizens. Key concepts include job creation, the circular flow of income, employment multipliers, and other important topics.

Learning Outcomes

- Participants will interpret demographic, occupation, and industry data.

- Participants will understand the importance of analyzing economic data.

- Participants will learn about basic vs. non-basic industry.

- Participants will discuss multiplier effects.

- Participants will become familiar with what information should be collected and reliable data sources.

Types of Data, Sources, and Analysis

Analyzing demographic, occupation, and industry data is required for community and economic development professionals to fully understand their local economy. Human nature dictates that assessing any community is essentially an exercise in compare and contrast. Two communities may have the same "feel" or visible similar economic activity even though they have widely disparate populations. Conversely, two communities with near identical populations may offer very different lifestyles and opportunities. There has never been as much readily available, high-quality data for those researching the nature of a place. Because of the dynamics just discussed, any one (or even two or three) static data point is insufficient for deep understanding of a place.

Compiling more data points tells a complete story when appraising a community. Trends and trajectory illustrate even more. Consider the Youngstown-Warren-Boardman OH-PA metropolitan statistical area (MSA) and the Fayetteville-Springdale-Rogers (Northwest Arkansas) MSAs. As of 2019, their populations were within one percent of each other. Comparing the two communities' economic data illustrates how the two could hardly be more different, although they have almost identical populations. Jobs (a 13% difference), household income (a 16% difference), and gross regional product (GRP) (a 31% difference) are a few examples of this point. This should not be surprising as Northwest Arkansas is one of the fastest growing MSAs in the country while Youngstown is in the midst of a decades-long decline.

When identifying catalyzing numbers, like the difference in the number of jobs, the multiplying effect on household income and GRP is evident. Those closely related fields can lead to the need for investigating such other secondary metrics as the number of business startups and local industry and occupation trends. Understanding (and certainly explaining) a place means understanding how it compares to its peers. But peers can come in many forms, as we've shown here. Start with a guiding primary statistic—like population—and look for significant deviations from peers. Then establish a new set of peers with a different primary statistic such as GRP and complete the same exercise. This "triangulated" approach will lead to interesting assumptions and insights as you seek to better understand a place and its economy. Case Study 2 at the end of this chapter will explain how to use this approach to redefine a community's peers.

Before a community can determine how it compares to its newfound peers, leaders must first analyze their demographic, occupation, and industry data. Federal, regional/state, local, university research centers and institutes, and subscription services are the five most reliable sources for this data. Specific sources within the demographic, occupation, and industry data categories will be outlined later in the chapter.

Demographic Data

Demographic data, typically sourced from the U.S. Census Bureau, offers insight into an area's individuals and households. The Decennial Census and annual American Community Survey (ACS) are the most recognized demographic data sources available to community and economic development professionals. Analyzing an area's demographic makeup enables community leaders to better understand their assets and opportunities. Population characteristics such as educational attainment, population by age and sex, and median household income are three commonly requested demographic data points.

Educational attainment refers to the percentage of an area's population, commonly 25 years or older, who have completed a particular level of education. For example, 87.7% of the U.S. population has earned a high school diploma or higher, while 31.5% hold a bachelor's degree or higher. Assessing an area's population by age and gender helps describe the current and future workforce. A higher than average median age, aging workforce, and declining birthrates may signal potential long-term challenges requiring local intervention. Median household income analysis is a valuable tool because it indicates how a community's household wealth compares against national, state, regional, and peer economies.

Occupation Data

Understanding occupation data is more important than ever in community and economic development, as an available skilled workforce increasingly ranks as the top critical site-selection factor. The U.S. Bureau of Labor Statistics (BLS) data enables community and economic development practitioners to evaluate the occupations and skills in their economy and then actively recruit relocation and expansion projects. To classify workers, BLS uses the Standard Occupation Classification (SOC) system, which allows the government and industry to produce similar data. Economic developers, elected officials, government employees, higher education institutions, job seekers, and employers are typical users of this data. *Major group, minor group, broad occupation,* and *detailed occupation* represent the four levels of the SOC system. Occupations are categorized into 23 major groups, containing 96 minor groups, 449 broad occupations, and 821 detailed occupations (*Standard Occupational Classification*, 2018). Occupations with similar skills or work activities are grouped at each of the four levels of hierarchy to facilitate comparisons. The most prominent occupation data used to analyze an economy are as follows:

- **Earnings:** describes the median hourly wage and annual mean wage by occupation for an area.

- **Employment:** the current and historical performance of an area's occupations gives insight into occupational growth or reduction and industries that support them. Projecting employment allows a community to demonstrate its available skills and leverage them to attract or retain employers.

- **Commuter patterns:** population is the number of people who reside in a political subdivision. But resident population has no greater impact on the economic activity or vibrancy of a place than daytime (worker) or visitor population. Determining the daily inflows and outflows of a community is a useful method to explain the presence or lack of certain types of businesses or the amount of economic activity. The On the Map tool (2019) provided by the Census Bureau Center for Economic Studies, determines this metric.

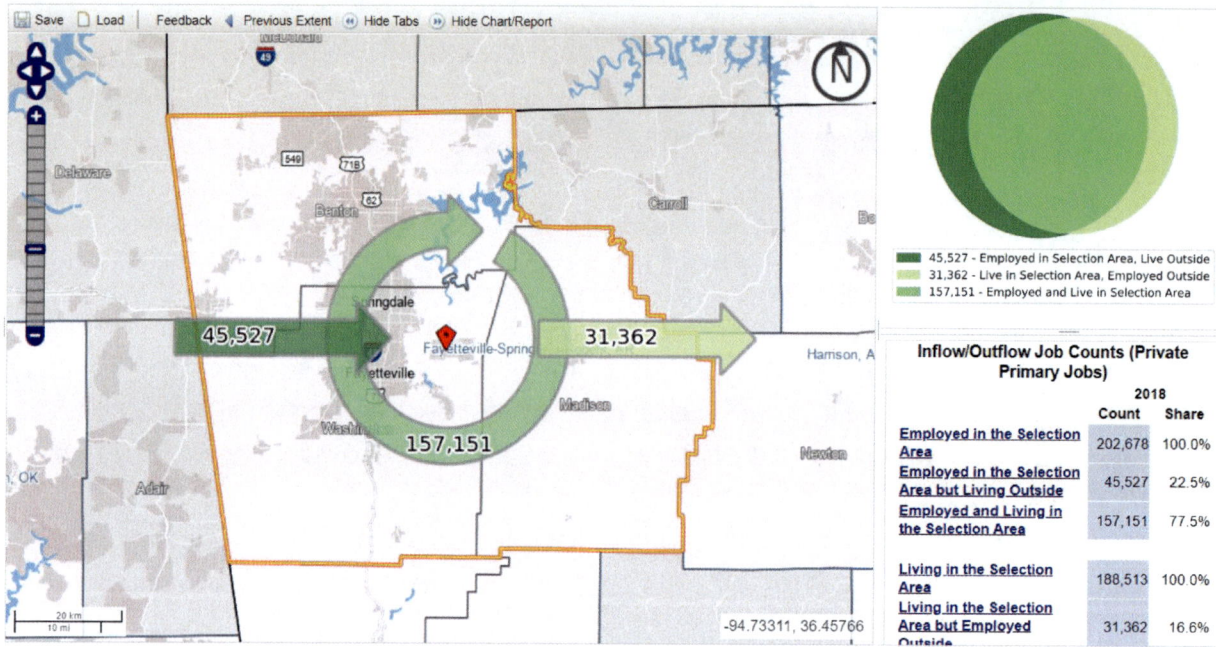

- **Laborshed:** explains the available workforce for a given occupation based on commuting patterns. The laborshed can vary depending on wages, other employment opportunities, transportation infrastructure, and other factors. Although employers are not traditionally a primary source for economic data, they can be helpful when compiling a database for further research. For instance, collecting the home zip codes of all employees for a particular industry, group of employers, or occupation would allow for the creation of a heat map detailing where area employees live.

- **Location quotient:** evaluates the relative employment concentration of a specific industry against the average employment of the same industry in a larger geography. A location quotient (LQ) greater than 1 indicates the area has a higher concentration of employment in an industry compared to the national average or another geography, while an LQ less than 1 indicates a below-average concentration (Minudri, July 17, 2020). LQs are calculated by dividing regional industry employment (r) by the national industry employment *(n)*.

- **Percent change:** this data point illustrates the increase or decrease in occupations over a period of time. Greater than average growth (an increase of 9% or more), average growth (an increase of 5% to 8%), less than average growth (an increase of 2% to 4%), nominal change (an increase or decrease of 1% or less), and decline (a decrease of 2% or more) are used to describe percent change (*Occupational employment projections to 2024*, 2015).

Industry Data

Partners involved in the community and economic development process cannot fully understand an economy without being familiar with industry data. Knowing what industries are expanding or contracting, for example, is critical. The most reliable source for industry level data is the U.S. Census Bureau, which allows community leaders to evaluate the industries in their economy and modify their job creation and retention strategy. The North American Industry Classification System (NAICS), created by the Census Bureau, groups industries that produce similar goods or services. NAICS uses a five-level hierarchy to classify twenty sectors of industry. These levels include sector (2-digit), subsector (3-digit), industry group (4-digit), NAICS industry (5-digit), and national industry (6-digit). Progressing through this hierarchy allows the user to analyze industries from the highest level down to the most detailed. The system currently employs 1,057 detailed 6-digit NAICS codes (North American Industry Classification System, 2019). The most relevant industry data analysis tools to evaluate the economy are as follows:

- **Earnings:** describes the average hourly wage and average weekly wage by industry for an area

- **Employment:** knowing the current and historical performance of an area's industries enables leaders to project future growth or decline for a particular industry as an industry's past indicates its expected outlook

- **Gross regional product:** similar to gross domestic product, gross regional product (GRP) measures the goods and services produced in a region. The size and regional nature of the local economy can make a place feel smaller or larger than its population.

- **Industry sector mix:** The Census Bureau Center for Economic Studies' On the Map tool allows users to determine the industry sector mix within a given community. Organized by NAICS code, this metric will break down the share of jobs by industry. When assessing the community, take note of the largest industries; by looking at previous year results you can see if those industries are growing or shrinking. Also, determine what desirable sectors are missing from the economy.

- **Location quotient:** denotes the relative industry concentration against the same industry in a larger geography. For example, Indiana has the highest manufacturing location quotient while Connecticut has the lowest construction location quotient.

- **Percent change:** illustrates the increase or decrease of an industry over a specific period of time.

- **Shift share:** explains which industries are competitive in an area by comparing expected and actual job growth against national growth. *Industrial mix effect, national growth effect, expected change,* and *regional competitive effect* are the four components of shift share. Industrial mix effect is an area's expected job change based on the industry's national growth or decline. National growth effect is the number of jobs an industry should add or lose based on the industry's national growth. Expected change is the specific job growth or decline within an area based on the national growth effect and the industry mix effect. The regional competitive effect indicates how much of an area's job change is caused by some competitive advantage (Minudri, February 27, 2020).

Economic Theories and Models

Three economic theories and models community leaders can use to better understand their economy are the *circular flow model, economic base theory,* and *input-output modeling*. The circular flow model demonstrates how money moves in and out of the economy. At the regional or even local level, money flows from employers to workers as wages and then back to employers as consumers purchase their products. This model also includes *inflows* (injections) and *outflows* (leakage) of money. Capital investments, government spending, and exports are examples of injections into the economy while imports, savings, and taxes exemplify leakage (Estevez, 2020). Although taxes are traditionally described as leakage, the recent creation and implementation of an internet sales tax by most states has led to the recapturing of tax dollars previously leaking through state and municipal boundaries with online sales. This illustrates how policy decisions can remedy leakage caused at the consumer level. Attracting upstream or downstream suppliers for existing employers as an economic development strategy is an example of how decision makers can inject money back into their economy and simultaneously reduce leakage at the employer level.

The economic base theory simplifies an area's economy into two industry employment types: basic and non-basic. Basic industries sell to nonresidents, bringing new dollars into the economy, while non-basic industries primarily sell to residents and capture dollars already in circulation. Manufacturers, information technology firms, and agricultural businesses are examples of basic industries. Restaurants, grocery stores, and banks are non-basic industries. Economic base theory contends attracting and retaining employers within the basic industry sector drives an area's economic growth (Watkins, n.d.). Ensuring there are diverse employers across the basic industry sector within an economy makes the region less susceptible to economic downturns because the area is less reliant on local dollars. However, non-basic industries are still critical, as these employers offer products and services required by residents and local businesses. Although a restaurant is traditionally considered a non-basic industry, if it expands to become a regional or even statewide tourism destination it would then likely be considered a basic industry. This example illustrates one challenge with the economic base theory in that overlap can occur between the basic and non-basic industries depending on the business cycle.

Input-output modeling is useful for predicting potential changes in the economic activity by measuring ripple effects on an area's economy triggered by changes in particular multipliers. Multiplier effects describe how a given change to an input causes a greater change in an output. *Sales, jobs,* and *earnings* are three of the most commonly used multipliers in several models. Sales multipliers show how a change in sales for a particular industry will impact sales in other industries. For instance, if $1 is added to a high performing cluster it may result in a sales multiplier of 6.0, meaning that $1 in this industry led to an additional $5 in regional sales. An employment (jobs) multiplier indicates how adding jobs in an industry will create jobs across other industries. Earnings multipliers show how adding employee compensation in an industry will create additional earnings in the economy.

Direct, indirect, and *induced* effects describe the results of these three groups of multiplier effects. Direct effects are the result of a primary activity being analyzed in an input-output model. Indirect effects are the regional supply chain purchases stemming from this initial activity. Induced effects demonstrate the consumer spending of employees within the business's supply chain (Wright, 2009). The following charts depict the addition of 500 automobile manufacturing jobs in the Youngstown, OH MSA and 350 data processing, hosting, and related services jobs to the Northwest Arkansas MSA. These examples will demonstrate direct, indirect, and induced effects within the earnings and jobs multipliers.

Effect on earnings from adding 350 jobs to Data Processing, Hosting, and Related Services

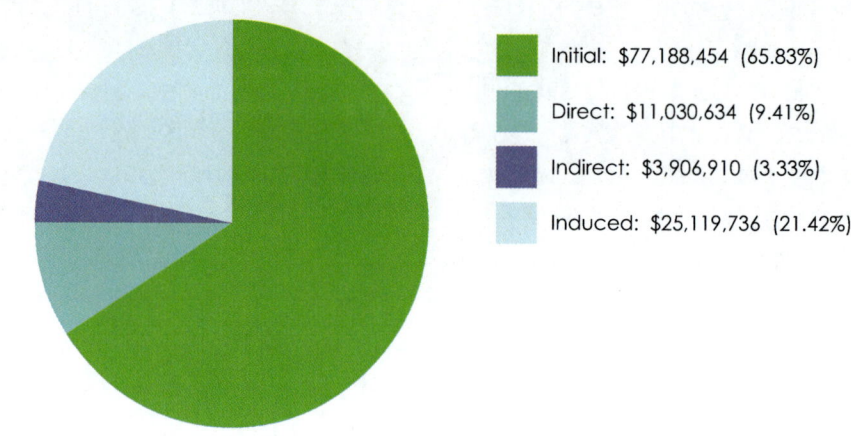

Initial: $77,188,454 (65.83%)
Direct: $11,030,634 (9.41%)
Indirect: $3,906,910 (3.33%)
Induced: $25,119,736 (21.42%)

$29,634,889.2 Initial	$9,241,931.6 Direct	$2,417,201.8 Indirect	$11,631,919.2 Induced
1.00 Multiplier	0.31 Multiplier	0.08 Multiplier	0.39 Multiplier

Effect on jobs from adding 350 jobs to Data Processing, Hosting, and Related Services

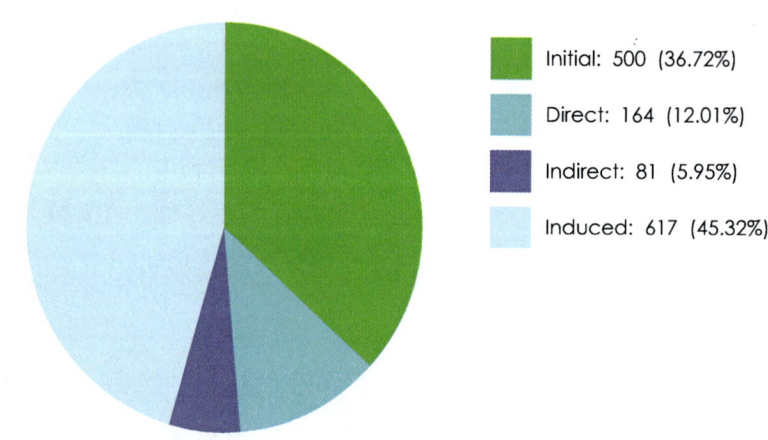

Initial: 500 (36.72%)
Direct: 164 (12.01%)
Indirect: 81 (5.95%)
Induced: 617 (45.32%)

350 Initial	202 Direct	51 Indirect	272 Induced
1.00 Multiplier	0.58 Multiplier	0.15 Multiplier	0.78 Multiplier

Effect on earnings from adding 500 jobs to Automobile Manufacturing

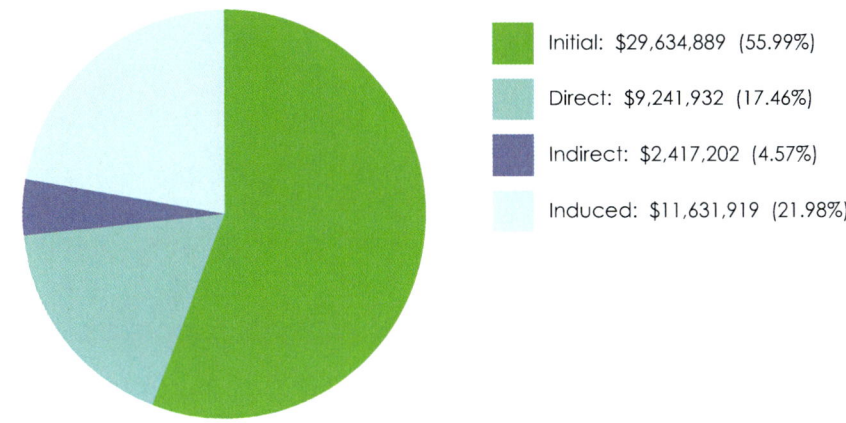

- Initial: $29,634,889 (55.99%)
- Direct: $9,241,932 (17.46%)
- Indirect: $2,417,202 (4.57%)
- Induced: $11,631,919 (21.98%)

$77,188,4	$11,030,6	$3,906,9	$25,119,7
54.3 Initial	34.2 Direct	10.1 Indirect	35.7 Induced
1.00 Multiplier	0.14 Multiplier	0.05 Multiplier	0.33 Multiplier

Effect on jobs from adding 500 jobs to Automobile Manufacturing

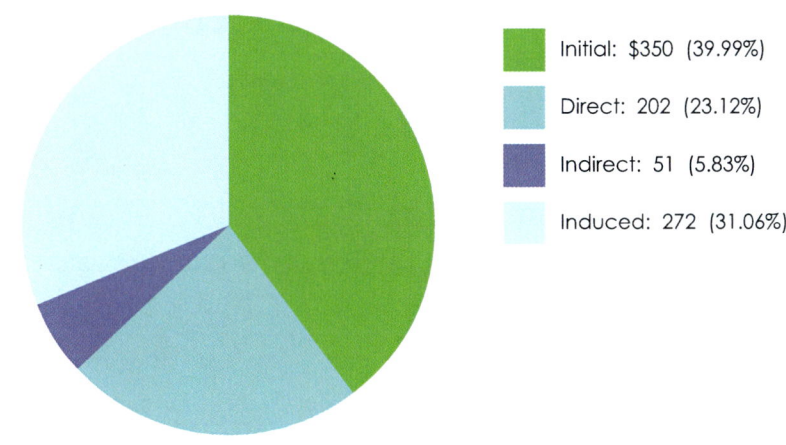

- Initial: $350 (39.99%)
- Direct: 202 (23.12%)
- Indirect: 51 (5.83%)
- Induced: 272 (31.06%)

500 Initial	164 Direct	81 Indirect	617 Induced
1.00 Multiplier	0.33 Multiplier	0.16 Multiplier	1.23 Multiplier

Data Sources

Accurate economic analysis requires reliable data sources. The following section details federal, regional/state, local, university research centers and institutes, and subscription service partners offering economic data. While this data source list is not exhaustive, it provides a solid foundation for collecting valuable information:

- **Federal:** Federal agencies including the Department of Commerce, Department of Labor, and Federal Reserve System report data on the national, regional, state, and metropolitan statistical area economies.
    - Census Bureau: reports data on population characteristics including race, education, income, poverty, housing, transportation, and local industry
    - Bureau of Economic Analysis: reports data on gross domestic product, consumer spending, international trade, and input-output multipliers
    - Bureau of Labor Statistics: reports data on inflation, prices, employment, compensation, and productivity
    - Federal Reserve economic research: The St. Louis Federal Reserve Bank, a private entity with the quasigovernmental Federal Reserve System, produces financial and economic data. Their FRED tool and research papers are available online.
    - Federal Deposit Insurance Corporation: reports financial data including bank deposit and market share reports.
- **Regional/state:** Regional and state organizations can be a great resource for local level economic data. The following are a few sources:
    - Economic Development Districts: EDDs collect information relevant to their jurisdiction's Comprehensive Economic Development Strategy, which helps guide the area's economic success. This data is useful for evaluating the regional and local economy.
    - Labor market information: Every state has an agency responsible for reporting labor market information, including local area unemployment statistics, occupational employment, employers by area, and wages by industry.
    - Sales tax collections: State departments of finance report state, county, and city sales tax data, which detail each respective area's retail sales and use tax collection receipts.
    - Utility providers: collect service area customer data that is useful for data analysis.

- **Local:** Many cities, counties, chambers of commerce, and economic development organizations are a useful source for collecting major employer, local sales tax, crime, and traffic data.
- **University research centers and institutes:** In addition to providing local jobs and training the future workforce, select higher education institutions offer data for public consumption. The following universities receive federal funding from the Department of Commerce and Department of Labor to provide economic data analysis tools and are the most well-known sources:
    - Harvard University: The Harvard Business School's Institute for Strategy and Competitiveness is home to the U.S. Cluster Mapping tool, which provides profiles of states, counties, and metropolitan statistical areas. These cluster profiles highlight regional concentrations of related industries.
    - Indiana University: The Indiana University's Kelley School of Business Indiana Business Research Center hosts StatsAmerica, which provides data profiles, maps, and other tools for economic development.
- **Subscription services:** Several private firms offer subscription-service data and analysis tools for community and economic development. The most popular systems are as follows:
    - Council for Community and Economic Research: C2ER is a membership organization that provides members with a regularly updated cost of living index, state economic development expenditures database, state business incentives database, and an economic diversity index.
    - Conway Data: Conway Analytics offers industry data about capital investments, job creation, and relocation and expansion leads.
    - Dun & Bradstreet: Through their D&B Data Cloud tool, Dun & Bradstreet provides company- and industry-specific data.
    - Economic Modeling Specialists, Inc: EMSI is a web-based tool that offers labor market information, job posting analytics, individual profile data, and compensation data.
    - Environmental Systems Research Institute: ESRI provides GIS mapping, location intelligence, and spatial data analytics software. ArcGIS, their most popular mapping and analytics tool, allows users to visualize economic and household data. The Business Analyst feature is especially beneficial for economic development.
    - IMPLAN: IMpact analysis for PLANning allows users to conduct valuable input-output modeling to evaluate the impact of an economic development project.

Case Study 1
Missing Kindergartners: The Economic Threat Hiding in Plain Sight

Public school enrollment in Arkansas has been slowly growing for more than the past decade. The state has generally added 1,000 or more students each year. Approximately 480,000 students attend public K–12 schools across the state. Over the next seven years, all of that growth, and possibly more, will be erased. While the state's overall population continues to slowly grow, the birthrate is falling at a record pace. Forecasts show that after the fall of 2021 public school enrollment will begin an increasingly rapid and sustained descent. And while the decline may officially begin in 2021, its origin goes back to 2008. In 2008, after several years of increasing birthrates, the number of births in Arkansas—and the entire nation—began to fall and have been decreasing ever since. The result is a public-school population whose largest cohort is in the 7th grade. The lower grades continue to decline with even smaller populations in the pipeline. This is not a short-term event. The state may experience brief upticks or flat enrollment for the next two or three years. But declining K–12 enrollment is the new normal, and it will have a serious effect on Arkansas's public policy and private economy.

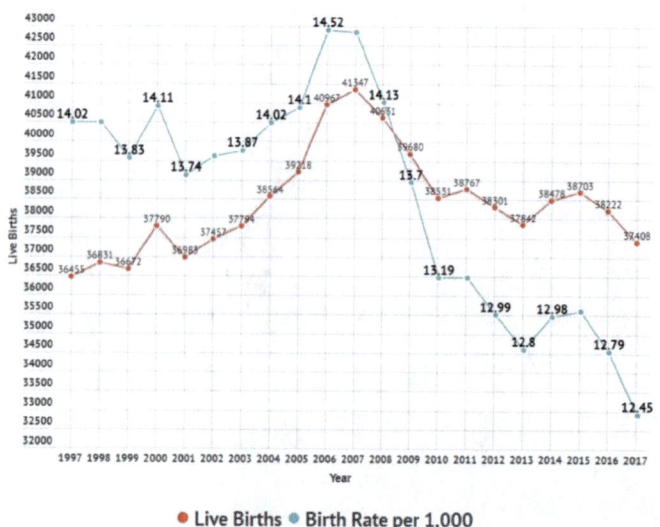

At least one factor driving the declining birthrate is good news. The single largest drop in the birthrate is among those aged 15–19. This reduction in teen pregnancy helps increase high school enrollment and graduation rates in the short term, because fewer pregnant teens means fewer students are dropping out of school. The other drivers are people getting married later in life and waiting longer into marriage to have their first child. The result is that in 2017 Arkansans gave birth to almost 4,000 fewer children than in 2007. That means in 2022, Arkansas will have almost 4,000 fewer kids in kindergarten than in the 10th grade. In fact, by the fall of 2021, each grade from 8th grade down to kindergarten will decrease in size according to the birthrate. The peak birthrate cohort will be in the 9th grade. K–12 enrollment in Arkansas will have peaked at around 481,000 students with both the century's largest (2007) and smallest (2017) birth year cohorts simultaneously enrolled. In the following five years, the state will likely lose more than 15,000 students.

These changes raise the obvious issue of funding and school finance. Arkansas spends about $9,000 per student per year on K–12 education. If that per-student number were to stay the same, the state could realize a savings of $350 million over that five-year period. Would lawmakers leave that money in the education bucket by raising per-student spending? Or will other priorities wait in the wings? Arkansas has a student-to-teacher ratio of 14:1. In a state with 15,000 fewer students, will districts make the decision to decrease the ratio? Or will they decrease the number of teachers? If public education in Arkansas were to shrink by tens of thousands of students and hundreds of millions of dollars, the impact will quickly spill over into other industries. The construction and bond finance businesses will definitely feel the effect—and then feel it again when this wave hits higher education. The same will be true for the hundreds, if not thousands, of vendors doing business with the more than 250 public school districts across the state.

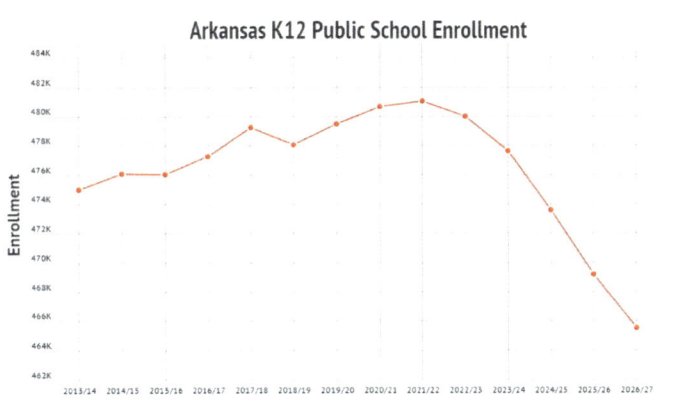

School District	% change in district enrollment 2013-2018	% change in KINDERGARTEN enrollment 2013-2018
Conway	+2.4%	-11%
Jonesboro	+15%	-3%
Springdale	+7%	-5%
Fort Smith	-1.5%	-16%
Fayetteville	+9.4%	+1.5%
Russellville	+2.9%	-14.2
Little Rock	-8.6%	-17%
Rogers	+5.7%	-1.8%

Arkansas's school districts are almost unimaginably diverse. Unlike many of the other demographic and economic shifts that have taken place in Arkansas, the falling birthrate and enrollment declines will be felt everywhere. Sustained declines in enrollment will eventually make their way through rural, urban, Delta, Ozark, large, small, poor, and affluent districts. From 2013 to 2018, 70% of districts have experienced a decline in kindergarten enrollment. More than half of Arkansas's growing school districts are experiencing a decline in enrollment in the lower grades. And those that aren't are seeing growth substantially slowed. A change this large will take time to prepare for and think through. This change creates enormous opportunities and challenges at the policy level. The same could be said for the private sector. How the state responds will affect everyone, regardless of generation.

Executive Summary / Key Takeaways

- K–12 public school enrollment will continue shrinking for the foreseeable future.

- Elected officials, departments of education, and school districts need to think strategically about how they will begin to reallocate budgets within K–12 education—or identify other priorities.

- Economies with a large construction, bond finance, and education employment base should prepare for the impact on employers by this change in school enrollment.

- Changes in K–12 enrollment will have a ripple effect on higher education institutions and a regional workforce pipeline.

Case Study 2

Dare to Compare. Leveraging Population and Gross Regional Product to Find Your Peer

Comparing places and their respective economies allows key decision makers to make informed decisions to move their communities forward. Analyzing community economic data can involve national, state, regional, county, and local data points. Although local level data is valuable, history or statute frequently complicate municipal boundaries, making them not especially useful when ranking. Regional—better defined as Metropolitan Statistical Area (MSA) level—data is the most relevant when comparing economic metrics. An MSA is a geographical region with a core population nucleus sharing close economies throughout the area. This case study will demonstrate how community and economic developers can use population and gross regional product data to redefine their peers by establishing where Arkansas and its two largest (MSAs) stack up nationally.

Figure 1

State - Population	City - Population
Iowa – 3.15M	San Diego – 3.33M
Nevada – 3.03M	Tampa – 3.09M
Arkansas – 3.01M	Denver – 2.88M
Mississippi – 2.99M	Baltimore – 2.80M
Kansas – 2.91M	St. Louis – 2.80M

Figure 1 shows that Arkansas's closest population peers at the state level are Nevada and Mississippi. And if Arkansas were a major city it would sit somewhere between Tampa and Denver. When making statewide decisions, community leaders need to understand Arkansas would only be the 18th largest MSA in the country. Yet the state is spread out over 10 to 20 times the land mass of either of those cities. At surface level, this exercise may seem humorous, but when trying to understand a community or region's economy, decision makers' first instinct is to ask how they compare to their competition. An immediate neighbor or a "rival" community in another region of the state will typically be the first candidate. Whether we're discussing policy or access to markets and talent, scale matters, so it is important everyone involved in the community and economic development process understands how to redefine "peers."

Figure 2

MSA – population rank	Population (2017)	Pop. Growth Rate 2010-2017	Gross Regional Product (GRP)	Per Capita GRP
Stockton, CA - #75	745,524	8.77%	$27B	$36,340
Cape Coral, FL - #76	739,224	19.47%	$28B	$37,813
Little Rock MSA - #77	**738,344**	**5.51%**	**$39B**	**$52,650**
Colorado Springs, CO - #78	723,878	12.12%	$33B	$45,139
Boise, ID - #79	709,845	15.13%	$34B	$47,339
Youngstown, OH - #103	541,926	-4.21%	$20B	$36,453
Northwest AR MSA - #104	**537,463**	**16.03%**	**$29B**	**$53,034**
Portland, ME - #105	532,083	3.5%	$32B	$60,409

Figures 2 and 3 illustrate how the Little Rock/North Little Rock/Conway MSA and the Fayetteville/Springdale/Rogers MSA compare to similar MSAs across the country. "Little Rock" or "Central Arkansas" MSA and the "Northwest Arkansas" MSA will be used for the remainder of the case study. As Northwest Arkansas has grown in size and influence, it's become fashionable for Arkansans—especially native Arkansans—to fixate on just how different these two places are. Out of the United States' 383 MSAs, Little Rock and Northwest Arkansas rank as the 77th and 104th largest. Beyond static population, when trying to identify a relevant peer, one of the key factors is rate of growth. Simply put, places (almost regardless of size) that are growing share a lot of traits and dynamics. The same could be said for those that are shrinking. While the Youngstown-Warren-Boardman OH-PA MSA has almost the exact same population as Northwest Arkansas, it will look and feel like a dramatically different place because its economy is a full one-third smaller and its population is in rapid decline.

No one familiar with Arkansas would be surprised to see the incredible rate of growth in Northwest Arkansas's population. It was the 14th fastest-growing MSA from 2010 to 2017, adding almost 75,000 people. Even though the Little Rock MSA grew at a much slower rate, however, it still added almost 40,000 people over the same time period. Again, scale matters. If each area maintains the same growth rate, the Little Rock MSA will remain the state's largest for another 22 years. At that time each MSA would have approximately 875,000 residents.

Figure 3

MSA - GRP rank	Gross Regional Product	Gross Regional Product Per Capita - rank
Tucson, AZ - #75	$39B	$38,165 - #297
Little Rock - #76	$39B	$52,650 - #129
Bakersfield, CA - #77	$37.3B	$41,808 - #253
Santa Rosa, CA - #93	$28.7B	$56,866 - #94
Northwest AR - #94	$28.5B	$53,034 - #123
Manchester, NH - #95	$28.4B	$69,424 – #37

Beyond population and growth rate, the final metric that helps determine true peers is gross regional product (GRP). It is the local equivalent of gross domestic product and measures the goods and services produced in an area. The size and regional nature of the local economy can make a place feel smaller or larger than its population. Also relevant is the per capita gross regional product. Places with a similar GRP will frequently have similar housing costs and retail options. It may surprise many that the GRP per capita in the Little Rock MSA and Northwest Arkansas MSA are within 1% of each other. Remember, though, that there are approximately 200,000 more residents in the Little Rock MSA. That's why you see leading retailers like Apple, Trader Joe's, and other with only one location in the state—and only in central Arkansas (Tampa also only has one Apple Store, by the way). Again, with retail—scale matters.

Northwest Arkansas's rate of economic growth is as impressive as its population growth. If both Northwest Arkansas and central Arkansas maintain their historic rates of GRP growth, they will be equal by that measure in 15 years. When ranking all of the MSAs in the country and by population, rate of growth, GRP, and GRP per capita, it becomes evident how Arkansas's two largest metro areas compare.

For the Little Rock MSA, such places as Knoxville, Tennessee, and Greenville, South Carolina match closely. For Northwest Arkansas, places such as Provo and Ogden, Utah, and Charleston, South Carolina, have meaningful similarities.

When analyzing the list of all 383 MSAs, however, it's possible that there are no two that could learn more from each other than Central Arkansas and Northwest Arkansas. This might surprise native Arkansans or those familiar with the two MSAs who know "how different" they are. What do you think? What places from around the country remind you of somewhere in your state? Where can the economies of your state look for ideas and direction?

Executive Summary / Key Takeaways

- By looking at population, growth rate, gross regional product (GRP), and per capita GRP we can identify our "peers" around the country.

- The state of Arkansas's population is approximately the same size as the Tampa MSA. Its economy is approximately the same size as San Antonio's.

- The Central Arkansas economy is more than a third larger than the Northwest Arkansas economy ($39B vs $28.5B).

- Northwest Arkansas is on pace to surpass Central Arkansas as the state's largest MSA in 22 years. It will be the state's largest economy in 15 years.

- Between 2010 and 2017, the Northwest Arkansas MSA added almost 75,000 new residents. During that same period the Little Rock MSA added almost 40,000.

- An "aspirational benchmark" for Central Arkansas is Des Moines, Iowa. "Aspirational benchmarks" for Northwest Arkansas are Boise, Idaho, and Santa Rosa, California. These MSAs share traits and have enviable metrics that could be matched by adopting intentional policies and economic growth strategies at the local level.

*These case studies were adapted from articles originally prepared for the *Talk Business & Politics* "Data Points" series. To follow the "Data Points" series visit www.TalkBusiness.net or search for #TBPDataPoints on social media.

References

Estevez, E. (2020, October 26). *Circular flow model.* Investopedia. https://www.investopedia.com/terms/circular-flow-of-income.asp

Minudri, I. (2020, February 27). *Understanding shift share.* EMSI: An Affiliate of Strada Education Network. https://www.economicmodeling.com/2020/02/27/understanding-shift-share-2/

Minudri, I. (2020, July 31). *Understanding location quotient.* EMSI: An Affiliate of Strada Education Network. https://www.economicmodeling.com/2020/02/03/understanding-location-quotient-2/

North American Industry Classification System. (2019). United States Census Bureau https://www.census.gov/naics/

Occupational employment projections to 2024. (2015, December 1). Monthly Labor Review, Bureau of Labor Statistics. https://www.bls.gov/opub/mlr/2015/article/occupational-employment-projections-to-2024.htm

On the map. (2019). Census Bureau Center for Economic Studies. https://onthemap.ces.census.gov/

Standard occupational classification. (2018). Bureau of Labor Statistics. https://www.bls.gov/soc/

Watkins, T. (n.d.). The economic base model. San Jose State University Department of Economics. https://www.sjsu.edu/faculty/watkins/base.htm

Wright, J. (2009, April 2). Input-output guidebook: A practical guide for regional economic impact analysis. (2020, November 19). EMSI: An Affiliate of Strada Education Network. https://www.economicmodeling.com/2009/04/02/input-output-guidebook-a-practical-guide-for-regional-economic-impact-analysis/

YEAR II

Building Entrepreneurial Communities
Jeff Standridge & Tiffany Henry

Business Attraction and Site Selection
Robert H. Pittman

Business Retention and Expansion
Dennis E. Williamson II

Community and Economic Development Finance
Toby Rittner

Quality of Place
Talicia Richardson & Claire Kolberg

Building Entrepreneurial Communities

Jeff D. Standridge, EdD & Tiffany Henry, MS

Entrepreneurship is strongly associated with economic growth. Discover what entrepreneurship is, what challenges startups face, and how to attract and keep these innovators. This session includes an analysis of what characteristics exist in an entrepreneurial community. Participants will rate their own community's level of entrepreneurship by assessing these same characteristics. The course will also provide tools communities can use to build extra capacity and to continue to build on that capacity.

Learning Outcomes

- Participants will discover what entrepreneurship entails.

- Participants will study the challenges startups face and how to attract and keep entrepreneurs.

- Participants will gain tools communities can use to foster entrepreneurship.

Entrepreneurs are the critical foundation of all thriving communities. Any amazing product, service, or movement that changed lives started with a wide-eyed entrepreneur at some point. Building something—anything, really—requires that spark from the one lonely soul who just could not tolerate the status quo another minute. The entrepreneur takes that first crucial step and says, "I can do this. I can solve this problem." That first determination begins a winding journey full of long hours, low (or no) wages, and no foreseeable finish line. For most, the motivation to begin this journey is not just the prospect of making money—entrepreneurs are motivated by notions of self-determination, not asking permission, and doing something meaningful.

The journey can be lonely, and the failure rate is high for entrepreneurs, particularly if their community does not have adequate resources or support measures available. An entrepreneur's community, which includes their physical place of being, personal and professional network, access to tools and information, and other amenities, is frequently referred to as an *entrepreneurial ecosystem*. An *ecosystem builder* is anyone who works to support and strengthen entrepreneurship in their community. This person may be a civic or business leader, educator, government official, or another form of community champion.

Why Does Entrepreneurship Matter?

The entrepreneurial spirit in the United States is thriving, and small businesses provide the foundation of the U.S. economy. From coffee shops and garages, to Main Street mom-and-pop shops, to ecommerce and cyberspace, entrepreneurs are everywhere you look when searching for the things that matter in your life. An entrepreneur's contribution to a community benefits everyone. Economic growth leads to lower unemployment and higher wages, which stimulates consumer spending. Gross Domestic Product (GDP) and tax revenues increase, resulting in reduced government borrowing and greater investment in schools, roads, and other public services. For every $1 in public money spent on downtown entrepreneurs, $26 in private funds were reinvested back into the community (McMahon, 2019).

In some circles, the word *entrepreneur* conjures a vision of a person who started a high-tech, high-growth enterprise. In this chapter, we consider an entrepreneur to be the founder of any venture big or small, urban or rural, technology-enabled or otherwise. We define *small business* as a venture having 500 employees or less with annual sales of $750,000 or less, and we define a *startup* as a new small business with high growth potential. The terms *startup* and *small business* will be used interchangeably throughout this chapter, but both refer to an entrepreneur's development of a new small company. In our experience building a venture ecosystem, we have discovered that supporting small and emerging businesses reaps the biggest social and economic rewards for the community, region, and state.

There are many reasons one may choose to start a business. Some people do so out of *necessity* while others seek *opportunities* to address an unmet market need or demand. Both necessity and opportunity entrepreneurs contribute to economic growth, whether they have one employee or one thousand. For many, being their own boss is tied to the identity and image of living the American Dream (Sappin, 2016). Starting a business allows the average person the opportunity to climb a few rungs on the economic ladder on their own terms.

How Does Entrepreneurship Impact a Community?

Small business owners know their communities and their neighbors. They show more concern for the local culture than outsiders or industry giants and have a vested interest in maintaining its vibrancy. As integral contributors to their community, entrepreneurial businesses improve society by providing locally made products and services; contributing to the tax base; providing jobs (perhaps for those who are unable to work elsewhere due to commuting or child care restraints); building community with customers and other businesses; and being actively involved beyond the scope of their business as a sponsor for a local sports team or sharing their knowledge and passion with students or local groups ("Best Countries for Business," 2018).

While American entrepreneurs have historically been white males, the rate of minority-, women-, and veteran-owned businesses is increasing (Benetrends Financial, 2019). Inclusive ecosystem building is a targeted approach to reduce barriers to equitable small business ownership and helps to support founders who are diverse in gender, age, race, religious or cultural beliefs, education, lifestyle, physical ability, or geographic location (Gines, 2019).

Why is Entrepreneurship Important in the United States?

More than 30 million small businesses are based in the United States and account for a staggering 99.9% of all U.S. businesses (*Small Business Profile*, 2018)! Many factors contribute to this high level of entrepreneurship. As a global superpower, the U.S. is a leader in technology (National Science Foundation, 2018) and innovation (*Global Innovation Index*, 2018). Venture capital, microfunding, angel investors, and a host of additional options offer a range of funding mechanisms. The country has a diverse population, and businesses enjoy greater freedom in decision making and product development than in many other countries (Abadi, 2018). The entrepreneurial environment is established and welcoming, and the continual expansion to accessible knowledge and ideas promises that entrepreneurs will continue to serve as the foundation to the U.S. economy.

Though most small businesses employ fewer than 20 people, their impact is significant. Entrepreneurs generate 44% of the economy, employ more than 47% of all U.S. workers, and account for 20% of overall job creation (Lauckner, 2020). The scope of entrepreneurialism in the U.S. is expansive. In 2016, more than 400,000 companies engaged in trade, and of those, 97% of importers and 98% of exporters were small or medium-sized enterprises. This translates to more than

$429 million in exports and nearly $618 million in imports. Not surprisingly, the U.S. is ranked as the top country for entrepreneurs by the Global Economic Development Index (*Global Entrepreneurship Index, 2018*) and *Inc.* (Abadi, 2018) and among the top three by *U.S. News and World Report* ("Entrepreneurship Rankings," 2020). We couldn't survive without them. Indeed, between 2009 and 2013, as the United States was slowly recovering from recession, 60% of new jobs were created by small businesses (Schmid, 2020). As magnified by the U.S. recession of 2020, it is vital that ecosystem builders continue to nurture and grow small businesses (Dunkelberg, 2018; *Small Business Profile*, 2018).

What Are Some Challenges to Entrepreneurship?

While becoming an entrepreneur has many benefits, it is not fail-proof. Many new businesses don't survive; only about half last for five or more years, and about a third will make it until their tenth year. New startups also are more sensitive to the economic environment and business cycles. The Great Recession of the early 2000s took a toll on the nation's entrepreneurial spirit, and recovery has been slow (Dinlersoz, 2018). The number of new business starts is at its lowest point since the late 1980s (Merkovich, 2019), compounded by the negative impact of COVID-19. For most entrepreneurs, however, the success of a new business is not tied to the status of the economy or even the presence of a global pandemic. Most (42%) startups fail because they created a product or service that no one wanted. This puts the business at a disadvantage from the start with the domino effect of inadequate cash flow and forced downsizing of employees (Schmid, 2020). Communities can help entrepreneurs in these critical early stages by helping with customer discovery and identifying product–market fit. Local ecosystem builders serve as trusted advisors, technical assistance providers, and oftentimes a source of encouragement. When a founder is feeling frustrated, ecosystem builders can remind them that entrepreneurs who had a previous business, whether successful or not, are 20–30% more likely to be successful with the next venture. Communities can also provide networking functions to encourage new relationships and opportunities for entrepreneurs to meet potential cofounders. These events serve as the catalyst for new ideas, new connections, and new possibilities. Entrepreneurship is hard work, which is why having a thriving ecosystem can help make or break the success of local small businesses.

What is an Entrepreneurial Ecosystem?

Critical to the success of entrepreneurship is a healthy entrepreneurial ecosystem. Formally defined as "a set of interdependent actors and factors coordinated in such a way that they enable productive entrepreneurship within a particular territory" (Stam & Spigel, 2016), entrepreneurial ecosystems provide a framework that makes available the resources necessary for entrepreneurs to start and grow their businesses.

Consider the metaphors of recipes and production to describe this ecosystem. Entrepreneurs try new combinations (i.e., different "ingredients") that create production recipes, the outputs resulting from a set of specific, distinct steps used to create the recipe. Entrepreneurship is the exercise of trying out the production recipes (Auerswald, 2015). Some are excellent and are used over and over; others are one-and-done. For example, a new small coffee/sandwich business may open at a train station to cater to rush hour commuters. The neighbors, however, take note and start stopping by, so the owner adds additional menu items. Recognizing the untapped market of the retirement facility down the block, the business adds card games and book clubs to the afternoon calendar. Trying different combinations to get to the best mix leads to a new production recipe. This "recipe" filled a food and social gap in the area, maximized use of the shop's resources, and added a productive new startup to the community.

There are many descriptions of what an entrepreneurial ecosystem is and how it is measured, but they all share several common elements (Isenber, 2011; Aspen Network of Development Entrepreneurs, 2013):

- **Human capital:** the availability of skilled and unskilled labor, high-school and college students, and training programs (a highly knowledgeable STEM-based workforce is even better)

- **Culture:** an environment that is tolerant of risk and mistakes and embraces innovation

- **Finance:** access to a range of funding options, including banks, government agencies, grants, venture capital, angels, and microloans

- **Markets:** domestic and international corporations, consumers, and distribution and marketing networks to create and fill demand

- **Policies:** established and reasonable tax rates, a regulatory framework, and incentives for doing business to create needed structure

- **Support:** infrastructure support (e.g., utilities, communications, transportation) and business support (e.g., legal and accounting advisers, technical advisors, mentors, incubators and accelerators).

The concept of an ecosystem to support entrepreneurs is still evolving. Although this approach has been used for more than twenty years, there are still areas that need to be more consistently established for a broader universal acceptance and implementation such as common measures, methods, terminology, and outcomes (Kauffman Foundation, 2018).

In addition to providing a starting point for new entrepreneurs, a strong ecosystem also helps to guide entrepreneurs as they navigate through new technologies, economies, and changes. An entrepreneur who starts a business out of necessity might shift direction to focus on the aspect of the business that offers the greatest potential to become an opportunity entrepreneur. The structure and support offered by an entrepreneurial ecosystem allows entrepreneurs to move from idea to realization. Lastly, strong ecosystems have frequent and consistent storytelling, shaping the narrative of a vibrant entrepreneurial environment while highlighting local successes. Storytelling creates momentum within a community and informs external stakeholders about progress and business opportunities. Clear and frequent messaging is vital to cultivating an environment that is open to risk-taking and innovation (Hodel & Meyers, 2017).

What Are the Four Pillars of Venture Ecosystem Building?

The four pillars that provide the structure and support for the rest of the entrepreneurial ecosystem are *talent, culture, community engagement,* and *capital*.

- **Talent:** A talented workforce is unquestionably the most important element in the ecosystem. This starts with the entrepreneurs themselves and extends to those who join them, not only the employees but also the mentors and advisors who guide them. Smart, ambitious, passionate people who are excited by risk and opportunity are attracted to the entrepreneurial culture, and they are central to the success of any business venture.

- **Culture:** Entrepreneurship requires the appetite to try something new and the bravery to continue even after failure. An entrepreneurial culture should embrace the same spirit of risk-taking and exploration. The culture should appreciate and celebrate people who are innovative, determined, confident, disciplined, and open-minded self-starters. This collaborative culture is reflected in the way municipal leaders make decisions, government officials set policies, and industry titans invest their time and resources. The culture of the wider ecosystem influences the startups within them.

- **Community engagement:** Common interests, goals, attitudes, and a sense of fellowship characterize communities. Entrepreneurial ecosystems epitomize and elevate the concept of community through a systemic approach to identifying, developing, funding, and sustaining entrepreneurship. This emphasis on interdependence across all factors in the system keeps the cycle alive and flourishing as new entrepreneurs are drawn to the community by the value of its talent, capital, and culture. Key actors in an engaged community are flagship enterprises, public institutions, local government, and the general public. Culture is what prompts an entrepreneur to start a business. Community engagement is what helps the business grow.

- **Capital:** Following closely behind talented human capital is financial capital. While some entrepreneurs are in the position to fund their own startups, most are not. Capital can be in the form of venture funding, SBA-backed commercial loans, CDFI microloans, or crowdsourced monies. Regardless of where the funds come from, an ecosystem must have capital available and be able to tell an entrepreneur where to find it.

Talent

One of the most exciting things about the entrepreneurial ecosystem is seeing the ingenuity and creativity as unique ideas come to life. What starts out as a thought becomes a tangible product or service that can become recognized and appreciated by ten or ten thousand users. Critical to this transformation is fostering an environment that attracts the right people to make the dream a reality.

The term *talent* is a great way to describe entrepreneurship because it takes a special gift to bring one's goals to life. Entrepreneurs also need an experienced and talented team to help fill the gaps in areas where their own skills may be lacking, such as record keeping or marketing. An ecosystem needs to support the development of both kinds of talent—the entrepreneurs themselves and the experts who help their companies grow.

Universities are some of the primary producers of entrepreneurial talent. Even though many famous entrepreneurs never graduated from college—including Steve Jobs, Bill Gates, and Mark Zuckerberg—more than 90% of tech founders have a college degree (Nayak & Farrington, n.d.). College isn't for everyone, but having a college in the local community contributes to a culture of learning, curiosity, and complex problem solving. In and of themselves, universities can serve as a hub for highly skilled and specialized talent. There is a circular effect as the brightest minds seek institutions that support their goals and, in turn, the institution produces graduate entrepreneurs who contribute to the community—there or elsewhere—providing opportunities for other great minds.

College is also the place where entrepreneurs often build lifelong relationships and meet potential partners, funders, and customers. Some universities serve in a boundary-spanning role. That is, they are influenced by the specific region and innovations of their location (for example, Minnesota is a hub for food and agriculture) and in turn provide reciprocal services such as incubators, technology transfer, research centers, and other collaborative opportunities. Though more scarce, there are also vibrant entrepreneurial university ecosystems. These universities are embedded within entrepreneurial regions and, through a lengthy process, develop the elements necessary to build an ecosystem and take on the many roles that help entrench it within the regional ecosystem (Malecki, 2018).

Though universities can be valuable assets in growing an entrepreneurial ecosystem, communities can begin fostering creativity and engineering skills far before students are college age. The natural curiosity of children can provide enough out-of-the-box thinking to completely change an industry. Gabby Goodwin was seven years old when she developed a unique double sided hair clip and founded her company, Gabby's Bows (Goodwin, n.d.). Her journey has been documented in the children's book *Gabby Invents the Perfect Hairbow*, which tells how an everyday frustration prompted the creation of a hair clip that is now worn by thousands of little girls. Sofia Overton was 11 years old when she participated in an event to pitch her Wise Pocket socks. Sofia took her product, designed with a pocket to snugly hold a cell phone, to the national stage when she pitched to the investors on "Shark Tank" (Overton, n.d.). There is no minimum age to become an entrepreneur, but the ecosystem must have the resources available to nurture young talent and connect them with tools that can help bring their business ideas to life.

An easy way for an ecosystem builder to foster young talent is to support art and creativity in the local classrooms. Research shows that children who show more imagination are better divergent thinkers and have higher creative thinking ability (Russ, 2018). Simple exposure to art and cultural institutions has tremendous benefits. Studies show that students who are exposed to museums and performing arts centers demonstrate significant and measurable differences displaying tolerance, empathy, educational memory, and critical thinking skills (Miller, 2013).

How Do Entrepreneurs Develop Talent within Their Businesses?

The first step to strengthening the ecosystem talent pillar is growing entrepreneurs. The second step is growing the talent that entrepreneurs need for their ventures to be successful. An entrepreneur's strategy to hire, retain, and develop a superior workforce is commonly referred to as *talent development*. It is most successful when the entrepreneur or manager (rather than a human resources representative or hiring firm) takes the lead in the recruitment and development process (Heathfield, 2019). This approach also helps leaders and their employees build a relationship, which can lead to a more engaged team and reduced turnover in the company (Bingham, n.d.).

A solid talent development plan should include clear vision, values, and goals to support the entrepreneur's objectives. One option is to complete a talent assessment of the company to identify any gaps in competencies or skills areas and to ensure there are diverse hiring practices from the very early stages of the startup. Talent development and assessment can occur through informal means like surveys or conversations or in official classes or workshops. The following items are simple strategies for an entrepreneur to nurture their workforce (Eyring, 2017; Olenski, 2015):

- provide mentorship and coaching
- offer regular assessments
- debrief after projects
- empower employee decision making
- cross-train across business units
- create networking opportunities
- earmark funding
- lead by example

Ecosystem builders can help their local entrepreneurs grow talent by connecting them to experienced mentors who can help young entrepreneurs develop much-needed self-confidence. Studies consistently demonstrate that having a mentor is instrumental to success in business. While only about half of small businesses survive past five years, 70% of businesses that have been mentored survive longer (Eugenio, 2016).

What is an Ecosystem Mentor?

Mentors provide insights on the entrepreneurship process and professional and personal support through the ups and downs of navigating that process. Access to several well-respected mentors is essential to entrepreneurial and ecosystem growth (Stam & Spigel, 2016). Ecosystem mentors have experience and knowledge valuable to startup founders and act as their advisors and confidants. Based on a survey of 33 entrepreneurial programs across the United States, researcher Jeffery Sanchez-Burks offers this definition of a mentor as someone who:

- inspires curiosity
- challenges assumptions and expectations
- guides through asking probing questions
- is honest and direct about what he or she doesn't know
- is eager to learn, along with the mentee (Brophy et al., 2017)

Mentors are a vital resource for entrepreneurs because they literally give away their experience! They know and understand the challenges founders face because they have been through it already. If a new crisis arises, they can call on a network of equally or differently qualified associates. Mentors understand what it takes to run a business and can help prioritize tasks and goals and offer a boost when things become overwhelming.

Talent development is a continuous process that includes exposing young people in the community to entrepreneurial thinking strategies, leveraging local university and educational resources to create entrepreneurs, and assisting entrepreneurs in their own quest to find and sustain a talented workforce. An ecosystem that attracts, develops, and retains robust talent is a place that can plant, incubate, and grow strong small businesses.

Culture

The second pillar needed to support a strong venture ecosystem is culture. For an ecosystem to successfully grow and support entrepreneurs, it must have a culture of innovation, collaboration, risk-taking, and curiosity. Starting a business is challenging in and of itself, and the likelihood of failure increases in the absence of an ecosystem with an experienced pool of talent, existing infrastructure of other businesses, networks, support services, and funding. For entrepreneurs to succeed, their community must support them. In addition to knowledge and capital, the community culture should demonstrate fortitude and recognize that failure and success go hand-in-hand. To promote networking and help navigate policy, entrepreneurs need strong connections and advocates at local, regional, state, and federal levels.

Ecosystem builders can help by creating opportunities to increase local businesses' visibility and connecting them with other entrepreneurs in the community. One way to do this is to identify resources and create a central portal for one-stop information shopping. Another key means of facilitating this connectivity is by ensuring a regular cadence of engaging events, programs, and activities that reinforce the entrepreneurial drumbeat. The venture scene must be event-driven. These events lead to "creative collisions" and unexpected connections that strengthen the venture ecosystem and reinforce the support for entrepreneurship within the "coalition of the willing" (entrepreneurs, investors, university representatives, community leaders, and others). When successful, this sort of event-driven approach combats one of an entrepreneur's greatest challenges—feeling that they are alone in their journey.

Another vital aspect of supporting an entrepreneurial culture is embracing and celebrating change. The most successful entrepreneurial cities have embraced change and willingly adapted to new circumstances. Cities with an entrepreneurial attitude view change as an opportunity and welcome the challenges that go with it. They know that business and economic growth benefits the greater good through more spending on education and health initiatives, and they actively participate in efforts to ensure that happens.

What Are Some Best Practices in the Development of an Entrepreneurial Culture?

The shaping of an organization's entrepreneurial culture is an intentional effort at every level. The nature of entrepreneurship suggests an open and dynamic culture. When the entrepreneurial mindset is encouraged in every business, industry, and organization of a local community, the innovative perspective will trickle out and influence the way local citizens view the community and make decisions. Here are some best practices for economic and community development leaders hoping to foster an entrepreneurial culture and influence community change from the inside out.

Hire entrepreneurs (Gerber, 2014). Research has shown that organizational leaders often look for people with qualities similar to their own. Community development organizations may have to widen their perspective and consider those with different skills and divergent thinking patterns to attract entrepreneurs. This makes good sense in an entrepreneurial environment because a community needs a talented workforce with drive, passion, and vision as they foster entrepreneurial activities to levels not previously imagined.

Be a learning organization (Social TrendSpotter, 2016). Training sessions are useful in their own way, but true entrepreneurial spirit comes from constant learning. This may occur in a class but is just as likely to take place from observations, discussions, failures, success, and a variety of other nontraditional methods. Learning organizations do not stop when they find a solution to a problem. Instead, they dig until they find the root cause and then solve that problem—in ten different ways!

Empower the team (Gerber, 2014). A leader puts a lot of time and thought into hiring decisions, so they shouldn't second-guess themselves once the new talent is on board. To embody an entrepreneurial spirit, team members should be given responsibilities and decision-making authority as well as accountability. Collaboration should be encouraged, and the team should know that everyone is a resource that contributes to the wealth of knowledge and experience of the organization (Howard, 2018).

Encourage sharing (Gerber, 2014; Social Trendspotter, 2016; Zwilling, 2017). Many organizations operate in silos, revealing only those aspects of their work necessary for a given project. Entrepreneurial culture is one of openness. Leaders should ask for recommendations and show team members that they are valued. Leaders should be candid that they don't know everything and that they value their team's wisdom. All team members should be comfortable generating ideas and having the voice to share them. It should be clear that both failures and successes contribute to the mission, and either outcome can lead to the next great innovation.

Prioritize diversity (Vaze, 2020; Hewlett, Marshall & Sherbin, 2013). The need for diverse teams has been a much-discussed topic in the last decade, but its importance cannot be overstated. Diversity can refer to inherent traits (what one is born with) as well as acquired characteristics (experience and perspective). Companies that encourage diversity contribute to a culture of innovation by providing an environment where different opinions are valued and employees have a high tolerance for risk.

How Can an Entrepreneurial Culture Be Created Naturally?

It is an ecosystem builder's responsibility to keep entrepreneurs front and center when developing community support. For the startup founder, the most rewarding feeling is watching an idea they have been nurturing come to fruition. For many entrepreneurs this reality transpires thanks to the generosity of funders, academic partners, or other entrepreneurial support organizations that are found in the ecosystem.

One connection that an ecosystem builder can help foster is between an entrepreneur and local funders. An ecosystem builder should identify common areas between the funding network and entrepreneurs and then provide opportunities for collision through events and activities. Entrepreneurs should not shy away from asking questions to ensure their goals and growth plan are in sync. Ecosystem builders can help entrepreneurs do their homework and come to the table with a clear and well-defined plan. As a result of this preparation, it is likely that founders and investors can work together to achieve a mutually rewarding experience.

Community Engagement

The third pillar in entrepreneurial ecosystem building is community engagement. Whereas an entrepreneurial culture entails creating an attitude of innovation and curiosity, community engagement is the actions that are sparked because of the culture. Engagement, in an ecosystem sense, is the interaction between entrepreneurs, employees, and other employers and community member that results in measurable improvement in desired outcomes for all parties. Engagement can be seen at all levels—from two entities forming a partnership to an advisor providing recommendations to an entrepreneur (Waugh & Miller. n.d.).

Community engagement is the collaborative efforts of groups of people related by geography, circumstance, or special interest to address their collective well-being. It involves partnerships and coalitions that can mobilize resources, influence systems and relationships, and serve as a catalyst for change. Pennsylvania State University's Center for Economic and Community Development describes it as a blend of science and art. The science reflects the many disciplines that contribute to the literature and conceptual development, including sociology, public policy, organizational development, psychology, anthropology and more. The art is seen in the understanding and sensitivity used to apply the science to the unique needs of each community and their specific engagement efforts (*What Is Community Engagement?*, n.d.).

Community engagement between entrepreneurs and civic and philanthropic groups can be done in many different ways. Examples include companies that participate in a day of service in their community, perhaps "adopting" a school or nonprofit and providing repair and clean-up services. Some organizations allow employees to donate an allotted amount of their work hours by volunteering with a nonprofit of their choosing. Businesses also provide support through donations to targeted initiatives and sponsorships of teams or events within their community. These individual and collective approaches build relationships and networks and contribute to a positive community culture regarding entrepreneurship. Employees pass on their skills and learn new skills in the process. These experiences offer great opportunities to experience teamwork in a different way. Morale is boosted, and pride in the company and community is reinforced (Gatty, n.d.), making it a win-win situation.

Community engagement is also demonstrated in the principal roles academic institutions play in entrepreneurial ecosystems. Colleges and universities provide a creative environment for students and faculty innovation and extend that role through collaborations with businesses and government. Increasingly, institutions are formalizing their commitment by offering degree programs in entrepreneurship that offer courses in developing networks, getting funding, and bringing an idea to market. Because learning entrepreneurialism and being an entrepreneur are two different things, these programs also typically provide opportunities to become involved in real-world entrepreneurial ventures.

What are Some Best Practices for Community Engagement in the Ecosystem?

As with any new initiative, it is important to have clear goals to achieve the highest level of engagement. Here are some best practices to help plan and design effective community engagement (Groundwork USA, n.d.; *Best Practices for Meaningful Community Engagement*, n.d.).

Identify relevant stakeholders. Be comprehensive and inclusive in recognizing local interest groups. Make a concerted effort to contact faith-based, cultural, racial, ethnic, and other underrepresented groups. Also, out of sight should not be out of mind—don't forget virtual and web-based groups.

Build trust. While working with many different constituents, it is important to be respectful of people's time, knowledge, and experience. Forming relationships and building inroads with communities will go a long way when trying to get an event or initiative off the ground. One must refrain from assumptions and judgment and remain open-minded and honest, particularly when people's businesses or ideas are on the line. No innovation or knowledge will be shared without trust.

Remove barriers to engagement. Consider where and how you will communicate. Accessibility to meetings or other gatherings by public transportation is important; so, too, is recognition that not everyone will have—or be comfortable providing—identification to enter a building. Provide materials or accommodations for different languages and physical impairments and give consideration to different levels of literacy; this includes use of jargon, technical language, and acronyms. Remember the needs of single parents who may have their children with them; offer child care and snacks as appropriate.

Offer different formats for engagement. Town halls and other public meetings are a great way to reach a large group of people at once, but they can become unruly and ineffective if the issue is controversial or a heated debate arises. Breaking out into smaller groups following the initial overview is more intimate and allows for greater discussion. Focus groups and workshops are also good forums in which to exchange information and gather input on issues. Smaller groups also allow opportunities to address language or other barriers to participation. Virtual opportunities can increase participation by allowing participants to engage at a time and location convenient to their schedule.

Don't discount opportunities for engagement that occur outside of formal gatherings. A community event is an ideal time to speak with people individually or in small groups where they feel more comfortable connecting. Other options include social events such as lunch with a councilperson or game night at a recreation center. Each table should include a community representative who can raise issues and facilitate discussions.

Establish ground rules. Let participants know everyone's roles and the goals for the interaction. Identify any nonnegotiable topics; this may include maintaining sponsor anonymity or withholding data outcomes before analysis is complete. Be sure to identify time limits for those who are more long-winded and allow time for those who may be more reticent to speak to feel comfortable enough to participate.

Do the right thing. When you bring people together to engage them, let them engage. Listen more than you speak and put yourself in their position to better understand their perspective. Be transparent about what can and cannot be achieved. Never bring people together under the pretense of being interested in their stories if you have no intention of incorporating their experiences. This defeats the goals of the ecosystem and negates any gains already achieved.

Community engagement is the thread that weaves together the components of the ecosystem and helps secure the four pillars in place. Entrepreneurs need the community to support their ventures, and communities need small businesses to create vibrant places to live, work, and play.

Capital

For any organization, funding keeps the fires burning bright, which is why the fourth pillar of entrepreneurial ecosystem building is capital. Entrepreneurs need seed money to buy equipment, find a work space, build a website, print business cards, and everything else needed to start the business. Some people rely on their own savings or ask close family and friends for this initial funding. For many, however, outside investors are the best source of funding, and this typically requires giving up part of the equity (Francis, n.d.; MyCorporation, 2018).

Once an entrepreneur has their venture set up and functioning, they need a steady cash flow to keep it operational. Utility costs, insurance, healthcare, taxes, salaries, and a host of other expenses must be paid. One burning question for entrepreneurs is whether or when should they pay themselves. There are different schools of thought on this. One approach is for them to view themselves as an employee or consultant, figure out their value, and include that amount in their business plan. Another view is to opt for a more modest salary, taking just what is needed to get by. Once the business becomes profitable, they can reevaluate to see if it makes sense for a raise. Some business owners may tie a salary increase to company growth; that is, if their business grows 20%, they take a 20% increase. It may seem counterintuitive to take money from the business one is working so hard to build, but an entrepreneur wouldn't ask someone else to work for free, and as such, they shouldn't necessarily put that burden on themselves (Siu, 2016; "Paying Yourself," n.d.). A community development leader can walk an entrepreneur through the options or connecting them with a local expert who can help address all their questions.

Entrepreneurs also need to give consideration to unexpected costs. A vehicle involved in an accident, customer refunds for lost or damaged shipments, or a flood in the basement could require a substantial outlay of costs. They should anticipate the cost of maintenance and upgrades to phones, computers, and software. If an entrepreneur has all of this covered and then some, they may be in a position to expand their business. While any costs associated with expansion should be offset by an increase in revenue, there may be a gap in timing between the outlay of expenditures and the realization of business growth. These scenarios must be considered in advance to avoid unsustainable cash flow restraints.

Achieving business goals requires funding, and a strong ecosystem provides these opportunities. Before approaching a potential funder, the founder should have a realistic valuation of the startup. Venture capital firms will want equity in the business, and one will need to determine how much he or she is willing to give up. Developing a strong business plan will help a business owner determine the worth of a startup three to five years out. Investors will appreciate the accurate representation, which also helps the entrepreneur know how much money to raise. While more may seem better, raising too much money may produce a poor return on investment (MyCorporation, 2018).

Worth noting again is the relationship aspect of entrepreneurship. Clearly funders are a critical part of an entrepreneur's success, but entrepreneurs should do their homework on venture capitalists and other possible funders to find a good fit. Top venture capital firms, which are very competitive, are often led by partners who themselves have been entrepreneurs, as opposed to lower-tier firms led by bankers (Endeavor Insight, 2015). This distinction is important because venture capitalists manage assets and bankers manage money. An ecosystem builder can help connect the entrepreneur to the source of capital that is best for them.

What Are Some Other Sources of Capital in an Ecosystem?

Capital comes in many forms, and it is important for ecosystem builders to know how each affects a business. Nondilutive sources of finance, such as debt capital, do not require that the entrepreneur give away any equity in the business. The most typical type of nondilutive funding is a loan. Debt capital must be repaid with interest at regular intervals over a defined period. This means that once a business owner has finished paying back the debt their liability is fulfilled. In some cases, the assumption of debt conveys tax benefits. Importantly, debt financing keeps full ownership of the business with the entrepreneur.

The big risk of taking on debt is that one must repay it regularly regardless of how successful (or unsuccessful) the business is. If a business takes on too much debt or misses payments, the valuation of the business can be affected. This may limit or prevent the opportunity for raising additional capital. Financing terms can also change if the debt has a variable interest rate or balloon payment (Cremades, 2018).

Other nondilutive sources of income are less common but worth noting. Licensing a project to a partner in the industry, using a royalty financing model, provides capital in exchange for a percentage of future revenues. Some businesses are eligible for tax credits, though these monies would be refunded or credited by the IRS after expenses are incurred. Grants also fall under this category, though these are generally limited to projects with an academic connection ("Non-dilutive," 2020).

Alternatively, an equity financing agreement requires that the entrepreneur give away partial ownership of his or her business in exchange for capital. This amount typically starts in the range of 15 to 25% but increases with each round of funding; it is possible that an investor may end up as an equal partner with half of the business. Equity financing offers significantly more capital than debt and, as previously discussed, brings in experienced investors who want the business to succeed. This comes, of course, at the expense of ownership share.

With any type of funding it is critical that all parties be clear on terms and expectations from the outset. The amount of capital needed and stage of business are key factors in determining best options. For example, nondilutive funding allows entrepreneurs to retain equity, but they may need to pay back the funds. If the funding need is so high that paying it back would be prohibitive, equity capital may be a better route. A thriving entrepreneurial community has the resources and the know-how to help entrepreneurs navigate the multitude of funding options.

How Can Entrepreneurs Build Scalable Ventures without Seeking Capital?

To restate our mantra: Entrepreneurial talent is key. Everyone on the business team has the ability to contribute or detract from the bottom line. When hiring, a business owner should make smart decisions and consider how each person can contribute to revenue even if he or she is not in a direct revenue-producing role. An administrative person might have experience negotiating, and people in tech roles can view the product from the customer's perspective to help ensure a positive experience. An ecosystem builder's network can also provide a mentor who has been in a similar position and can offer their insights.

A community developer need not have a background in finance to suggest simple ways an entrepreneur can save cash and self-fund their venture. By remaining frugal where one can, funds can be directed where they will have the greatest impact. Entrepreneurs can pack a peanut butter and jelly sandwich for their own lunch but take clients somewhere nice. Business owners can skip the nonessentials and invest in their product or service. A community development leader can share these tips with local entrepreneurs or facilitate a barter system to provide opportunities to entrepreneurs to trade their talent and skills. For example, conference volunteers typically attend those events for free. If an entrepreneur signs up for registration duty, they can attend the event and receive the added benefit of meeting the key players in their industry. (Baydin, 2020; Zwilling, 2016)

Start Where You Are

The four pillars of ecosystem building consist of talent, culture, community engagement, and capital. Tapping into an existing infrastructure is one thing, but what if the community isn't quite there yet? Understanding the assets, aspirations, and community gaps is a crucial first step. Smaller cities and towns may live in the shadow of metropolitan areas, but they can still become an entrepreneurial hub by building on their own unique strengths and resources.

How Does a Community Assess Where They Are?

For ecosystem builders to know where to start in evaluating their current community assets, they must take stock of what they can offer to support entrepreneurship and what they have yet to develop. One way to do this is to conduct a market analysis of the community (*Supporting Entrepreneurship*, 2011). This type of in-depth study identifies types and sizes of existing businesses, potential customers, and market needs. Although market analyses typically include a section on competitors, in the case of assessing a community for its ability to become a hub for entrepreneurs, the competitor analysis could be an extension of the business analysis. A community development leader should have knowledge about the local business landscape, which will provide insight about their volume, employees, services provided, support services, and other critical information. This helps identify strengths and gaps in a potential ecosystem. It also helps identify what level of entrepreneurship already exists.

An important part of a market analysis is to identify any barriers or obstacles to starting a business, including policies and regulations. Government regulations can make or break a welcoming community. An entrepreneur-friendly local government directly influences how businesses operate in their community, and they can work to encourage change at the regional or state level. For example, registering as a business and completing necessary forms and paperwork is a time-consuming effort. Local governments can simplify their regulations for starting a business and seek input from existing businesses to identify and eliminate confusing or superfluous steps. An online portal that includes necessary forms, contact information, FAQs, and other resources will streamline the process and let entrepreneurs know that the government is working toward their success, not detracting from it.

Many entrepreneurs start out working or distributing products from their home. Zoning codes should allow for the existence of combined-use business–residential properties. For businesses located outside the home, an inviting environment will draw both entrepreneurs and customers. Walkable business districts encourage residents and visitors to spend time in the area. This creates greater tax revenue per square foot than other types of development. Local government and businesses can do their part by slowing traffic, adding benches, and beautifying the area (Quednau, 2016).

Policy- and decision-makers are also instrumental figures in local networks. These representatives should demonstrate their commitment to development in their community and region by working to attract not only entrepreneurs but such key elements of the infrastructure as STEM education and talent development programs. If the area is home to a university, strong links and open lines of communication to the community should be facilitated. If not, encouraging a strong anchor business whose product and values are aligned with the region should be a priority. This high-level presence demonstrates mutual commitment from the business and community to support one another and the development of the region.

In addition to politicians, support from other key figures such as CEOs, lawyers, investors, and the local press can be used to the community's advantage.

Sharing resources, hosting events, and providing coverage of the contributions of local startups gives a clear indication that entrepreneurial culture is (or will be) reflective of all facets of the community. Similarly, creating opportunities for entrepreneurs to share their stories, successes, and failures with others who have had similar experiences is a critical component of information sharing that is core to entrepreneurial practice (Edward Lowe Foundation, 2020).

What Is the First Step in Building an Entrepreneurial Ecosystem?

Providing entrepreneurial programming and networking events are the quickest way to jumpstart an entrepreneurial ecosystem. These events offer opportunities to share ideas and best practices or to get help overcoming an obstacle a community might be facing. These groups offer professional and social networking, strategy and marketing insights, recruiting opportunities, and introduction to potential funders. Connections and opportunities also can be found through alumni organizations, social and religious organizations, and government programs. Additionally, there are any number of professional associations representing different industries, membership groups, and causes that have local chapters throughout the country. These groups host professional and social events and many offer speaking or award opportunities as a benefit of membership. Joining an online community offers the added advantage of bridging distance and offers the flexibility of nonsynchronous activity.

Having a network is important to all professionals (and all people). Entrepreneurs, in particular, need a strong network because they start from the ground up. Someone who works for or develops a new idea for a Fortune 500 company has a built-in network. They can call on supervisors, support staff, colleagues, partners, and the tens or hundreds of others who interact with the many facets of the business. A startup may consist of only one or two people for the first few years, but they still need a support infrastructure, and networking is the way to build it.

As entrepreneurs share their ideas with friends and family, they are likely to hear comments like "My sister-in-law works with a guy who used to do that—I'll give you his number." This is the beginning of the professional network: friends of friends, former coworkers and classmates, neighbors' in-laws, and the person in the next seat at National Entrepreneurs' Day. Community developers can create opportunities for entrepreneurs to form relationships that are mutually beneficial.

What Are Some of the Best Practices Involved in Creating a Thriving Network of Entrepreneurs?

As a community development leader, you likely already have the connections and relationships required to build a solid network of entrepreneurs. Here are a few steps you can take to help identify key assets to creating a vibrant entrepreneurial network.

Have a plan. Developing your professional contacts is a must, and networking is how it is done. To make the most of your efforts, take time to develop a plan. Consider your goals and what you want to achieve. Think about which entrepreneurs you desire to know and the best opportunities to meet them. Look for opportunities to connect others within your ecosystem, including entrepreneurial competitors to maintain neutrality and inclusivity. Also think about your role in the community and how you can give back in a meaningful way that is important to you.

Be intentional and selective. Time is the most valuable asset an ecosystem builder has. Local events are important, but don't let mileage dictate your networking circle. Become familiar with organizations in your region and the types of events they host. Take advantage of sources that provide calendars of events weeks in advance so you can schedule time for networking.

Networking is two-way. Finding like-minded others who support entrepreneurship is critical to the growth and success of the ecosystem. Equally important is being a source of support for others. When looking for events that will help grow your network, also look for opportunities to be of service. You might mentor a college student or give a presentation on an area of expertise at a library or senior center. Sponsoring a sports team or town event is a great way to show support and generate some publicity. Think about what you hope to gain from networking and offer that same opportunity to someone else through an introduction or problem-solving advice.

Smaller communities and towns should not be deterred from encouraging entrepreneurship based on their size or location. Community leaders can reach out to local entrepreneurs and their own networks to identify needs and opportunities, and to local businesses to build relationships and expand networks. The effort that communities invest is returned through the positive ripple effect in the economy and region ("Networking," n.d.; Wither, 2020; Oracles, 2017; Rittscher, 2012; Young Entrepreneur Council, 2018).

What are Some Other Types of Programs a Community Can Host to Encourage Entrepreneurship?

In addition to joining a group or attending an event, communities can create their own workshops to encourage entrepreneurship. Business owners can offer a class on topics of interest to startups, such as accounting or marketing, or they can join forces with a university to host a conference on a range of topics. Any community can take part in increasingly popular annual events such as Global Entrepreneur Week, Startup Week, and Small Business Saturday.

The range and diversity of the programs and events available in ecosystems shows the commitment of their entrepreneurial infrastructure. Although the culture of the communities and entrepreneurial ecosystems are unique to each region, events and programs shared across these and other systems can serve as a framework for budding systems. Consider the following options when developing a support structure within your entrepreneurial community.

Don't go it alone. A required characteristic of an entrepreneurial ecosystem is community-wide support from existing small and large businesses; local, regional, and state governments; financial institutions; and other entrepreneurs, just to name a few. These ecosystem members come with a wealth of knowledge and may be waiting for an invitation to share it. Who better to talk about tax issues than an accountant? A tutorial from a city government representative can save someone a day or more trying to decipher required forms and paperwork. National and international support organizations such as the Kauffman Foundation, Techstars, StartupNation, and Pipeline are great resources for identifying issues—and solutions—relevant to entrepreneurs.

No need to reinvent the wheel. There are literally hundreds of programs and events hosted every day by different groups, from offering personal advice or business information, to startup weekends and boot camps. Chambers of commerce, universities, associations, libraries, meetup groups, and dozens of other organizations post calendars of events a few weeks or months in advance. These represent different formats, times of day, duration, venues, and topics, providing something for everyone. Some groups are informal and meet for coffee while others host more structured meetings and events. There are also state-level and national programs, such as 1 Million Cups, directed at entrepreneurial growth.

Offer breadth and depth. As seen in these examples, programs are available on virtually every topic an entrepreneur might need to learn or develop, from creating a business plan to finding capital to marketing and networking to scaling a business and going public. And speaking of virtually, offerings such as webinars,

MOOCs (massive open online courses), TED Talks, LinkedIn groups, and other online opportunities provide information on both broad and niche issues.

Collaborate with entrepreneurs. While family and friends are great sources of support for an entrepreneur, knowing others who have successfully faced similar challenges can make all the difference in bringing an idea to reality. Events hosted by entrepreneurs, for entrepreneurs, are a must for all ecosystems. No one knows better the joy of acquiring a first round of funding or the despair of another prototype disappointment than those who have lived the experience. Events pairing entrepreneurs combine learning and networking opportunities and, because many angel investors are entrepreneurs in their local community, the potential for financing.

Show and tell. The events noted here focus on programs that provide information to entrepreneurs. However, as every entrepreneur knows, often jumping in and doing something firsthand enhances the experience. In addition to being an audience member, community development leaders can also create awareness and interest by participating at various events. Speaking at schools or community events promotes entrepreneurship and community building. Additionally, many groups offer awards for different entrepreneurial-related efforts. Self-nominating is a great way to promote an innovation with the added benefit of networking at the award ceremony. Entrepreneurs who may not be ready to submit their own projects can show their support for others by nominating someone else.

How Can You Leverage Your Community's Unique Advantages?

Looking inward also compels communities to focus on the needs of their own region. Communities recognize what holds them back from being competitive or otherwise limits their ability to showcase their resources. The members of a community are its lifeblood and are aware of its imperfections and potential, and they are vested in creating opportunities for themselves, their children, and their neighbors. It is this intensive, intimate knowledge that distinguishes one community from another, and it is these unique attributes that each community should leverage.

Does your ecosystem need help identifying world-class assets? Start by looking at the history of the region and the industries that contributed to its growth. This can help leaders understand their community's value. It is important to look beyond business contributions. Many of the emerging ecosystems are in cities known for their relaxed lifestyle and culture. Good schools, sustainability, parks and recreation, and arts contribute to a location's appeal. Community attributes such as creativity, generosity, and patience are valued and should be promoted as assets.

Building an entrepreneurial ecosystem is vital for communities to stay competitive and economically viable in the 21st century. But as the old adage goes, ecosystems aren't built in a day. It can take years before the seeds planted in the ecosystem begin to sprout and take root; however, the hard work done today will reap a harvest of innovation and entrepreneurship for generations to come.

Case Study
The Conductor: Founded on Four Pillars

One of the most successful examples of growing and supporting the four pillars of entrepreneurial ecosystem building (talent, culture, community engagement, and capital) is the creation of the Conductor in Conway, Arkansas. While the organization officially launched in November 2016, the journey began three years prior with a committee of committed "community change agents" convened by then-Chamber of Commerce Board Chair, Dr. Jeff D. Standridge. Standridge also served as an executive with data and technology firm Acxiom Corporation at the time. This committee spent nine months interviewing entrepreneurs (both successful and unsuccessful) and entrepreneurial ecosystem builders around the country as well as around the state of Arkansas. In late 2014, Standridge convened a summit of committee members, local community leaders, college and university presidents, as well as key ecosystem builders from across the state to present the committee's findings.

A featured guest at this summit was Jeff Amerine, founder of Startup Junkie Consulting (SJC). Amerine had been a respected leader in the entrepreneurial space for more than a decade, having previously worked as the Associate Vice Provost, Research and Economic Development, and Director of Technology Ventures at the University of Arkansas. He has held senior leadership positions in nine startups and three Fortune 500 companies and has made more than 90 early-stage investments into new ventures and small businesses either directly or through the funds he manages.

Following the event, a conversation developed between Amerine and then-University of Central Arkansas (UCA) president Tom Courtway. Courtway recognized the role a university plays in developing young innovative talent, particularly that entrepreneurship is the key to prepare local students for the future knowledge economy—and also a great strategy to keep UCA graduates in Conway. In his quest to explore the community capacity for building an entrepreneurial ecosystem, Courtway contracted with SJC to conduct a seven-month feasibility study of the region. Included in the assessment committee were the Conway mayor, leaders from the Conway Chamber of Commerce and Economic Development Corporation, college and university faculty, and Conway Corporation, a local utility company.

At the conclusion of the study, SJC reported that Conway was at a pivotal moment in time, prime for entrepreneurial support, partly because of the strong collaboration and demonstrated unity between all of the project constituents. Amerine and his team recommended that UCA begin an initiative focused on entrepreneurial development that would serve to increase research and commercialization opportunities for the faculty, provide entrepreneurial opportunity for the students, and connect the university to the community through large events, training, and programming. An eventual agreement between UCA and SJC resulted in a public–private partnership, and in November 2016 the Conductor was born.

Coincidentally, Standridge, himself an accomplished entrepreneur—having led established businesses and startup companies in North and South America, Europe, Asia, and the Middle East—had retired from his role at Acxiom. Because of his deep roots in the community and proven entrepreneurial acumen, he was brought on board as the Conductor's first managing director. With a mission to *Empower and Inspire Innovators, Entrepreneurs, and Makers*, the Conductor started working right away with a focus on developing the four pillars of talent, culture, community engagement, and capital in Conway. This is done through one-on-one coaching and consulting, technical assistance workshops, networking events, startup promotion activities, and student development programming. Because of the partnership with UCA, all of the Conductor offerings are provided free of charge.

Within the first year, the Conductor surpassed 1,000 engagements through individual meetings and group events. In 2017, because of this success, UCA expanded the contract to include a makerspace to provide innovation and prototyping experience and use of 3D printers, laser engraving, woodworking tools, and other equipment that supports creativity and discovery. Four years after opening its doors, the Conductor has served more than 10,000 people and expanded its offerings from the city of Conway to a 12-county region in central Arkansas. In 2019, Conway Corporation announced the acquisition of the former City Hall in downtown Conway and a planned multimillion-dollar renovation that will create a permanent home for the Conductor in the Arnold Innovation Center, named after retired Conway Corporation CEO Richie Arnold.

The four pillars of ecosystem building remain the priority of all Conductor activities, which are demonstrated as follows:

Talent

The Conductor is a key driver of entrepreneurial talent development in central Arkansas. Utilizing two outbound educators, the Conductor engages with school-aged children on projects involving coding, robotics, art, and sustainability. Specific trainings have been held with such groups as the Girl Scouts on pitching their cookies and conducting customer discovery. The Conductor has partnered with a local marketing agency to host a high school brand camp and also worked with a large healthcare system for a university-level Health Sciences Entrepreneurship Bootcamp. The makerspace also holds trainings for all ages and has welcomed many field trip groups.

Culture

Utilizing its venture ecosystem curriculum, the Conductor works with community leaders to help foster a culture of entrepreneurship and innovative thinking through an asset-based approach to identifying existing startup resources using the four-pillar approach. The Conductor also works with startups and established businesses on strategic planning to help promote a workplace that values and supports entrepreneurial thinking. These business leaders often incorporate the skills and lessons learned into their additional community responsibilities. Developing an entrepreneurial culture both within a startup and in a community are frequent topics of one-on-one consultations.

Community Engagement

The Conductor hosts regular networking events and workshops that are designed to encourage relationships and new learning opportunities. Activities include fireside chats with established community leaders on their professional journeys, stories from startup founders on their lessons learned, and pitch events sponsored by local banks or businesses. Events are inclusive and welcoming, often hosted in partnership with other local organizations. The Conductor has also begun advocating for policies that reduce barriers to entrepreneurship by working closely with government and civic leaders and providing informational resources.

Capital

Access to capital is commonly referenced as one of the biggest barriers to entrepreneurship. The Conductor hosts regular angel investor meetings to connect members with early stage companies. It also partnered with a national resource provider to facilitate 0% interest loans to underserved rural entrepreneurs. Technical assistance support includes budgeting and finance guidance, as well as communicating often-overlooked topics such as the importance of

> forming a relationship with a local banker. Pitch events are another pathway to capital infusion for a startup founder.
>
> An organization does not need to be an official entrepreneurial support group to foster the four pillars of ecosystem building. As the success of the Conductor has shown, all one needs is an attitude of collaboration, a spirit of trust, and the intrinsic drive to empower and inspire innovators, entrepreneurs, and makers in the local community.

This chapter was adapted with permission from *Creating Startup Junkies: Building Sustainable Venture Ecosystems in Unexpected Places* (Amerine & Standridge, 2021).

References

Abadi, M. (2018, October 17). 25 best countries in the world to start a business. *Business Insider*. https://www.inc.com/business-insider/25-best-countries-in-the-world-to-start-a-business.html

Amerine, J. & Standridge, J.D. (2021). *Creating startup junkies: Building sustainable venture ecosystems in unexpected places.* Highpoint Executive Publishing.

Aspen Network of Development Entrepreneurs. (2013, December). *Entrepreneurial ecosystem diagnostic toolkit.* Aspen Institute. https://assets.aspeninstitute.org/content/uploads/files/content/docs/pubs/FINAL%20Ecosystem%20Toolkit%20Draft_print%20version.pdf

Auerswald, P.P. (2015, October). *Enabling entrepreneurial ecosystems.* Kauffman Foundation. https://www.kauffman.org/-/media/kauffman_org/research-reports-and-covers/2015/10/enabling_entrepreneurial_ecosystems.pdf

Baydin, A. (2020). How to build a scalable tech business without VC funding. *Inc.*. https://www.inc.com/alex-baydin/how-to-build-a-scalable-tech-business-without-vc-funding.html

Benetrends Financial. (2019, March 18). *American minority business owership: A look at the stats.* https://www.benetrends.com/blog/american-minority-business-ownership-a-look-at-the-stats

Best countries for business 2018. (2018). *Forbes*. https://www.forbes.com/places/united-states/#288fbe2b236d

Best practices for meaningful community engagement: Tips for engaging historically underrepresented populations in visioning and planning. (n.d.). Groundwork USA. https://groundworkusa.org/wp-content/uploads/2018/03/GWUSA_Best-Practices-for-Meaningful-Community-Engagement-Tip-Sheet.pdf

Bingham, T. (n.d.). Developing talent drives engagement and business success. *Future of Business and Tech*. http://www.futureofbusinessandtech.com/education-and-careers/developing-talent-drives-engagement-and-business-success

Brophy, D., Jenson, T., Kagan, E., Milovac, M. & Sanchez-Burks, J. (2017, November). *Mentoring in startup ecosystems.* University of Michigan Ross School of Business. https://deepblue.lib.umich.edu/bitstream/handle/2027.42/139028/1376_Sanchez-Burks.pdf?sequence=1&isAllowed=y

Community Places. (n.d.). *Community planning toolkit: Community engagement.* https://www.communityplanningtoolkit.org/sites/default/files/Engagement.pdf

Cremades, A. (2018, August 19). Debt vs. equity financing: pros and cons for entrepreneurs. *Forbes*. https://www.forbes.com/sites/alejandrocremades/2018/08/19/debt-vs-equity-financinpros-and-cons-for-entrepreneurs/#25f675f46900

Dinlersoz, E. (2018, February 8). *Business formation statistics: A new Census Bureau product that takes the pulse of early-stage U.S. business activity.* United States Census Bureau. https://www.census.gov/newsroom/blogs/research-matters/2018/02/bfs.html

Dunkelberg, W. (2018, December 20). Growth and full employment on Main Street. *Forbes*. Retrieved from https://www.forbes.com/sites/williamdunkelberg/2018/12/20/growth-and-full-employment-on-main-street/?sh=428189523efd

Edward Lowe Foundation. (2020). *Building entrepreneurial communities.* Natural Capitalism Solutions. https://www.natcapsolutions.org/LASER/LASER_Building-Entrepreneurial-Communities.pdf

Endeavor Insight. (2015, December 2). Entrepreneurial experience separates top VCs from other investors. *TechCrunch*. http://www.ecosysteminsights.org/entrepreneurial-experience-supports-the-best-vcs-from-other-investors/

Entrepreneurship rankings. (2020). *U.S. News*. https://www.usnews.com/news/best-countries/entrepreneurship-rankings

Eugenio, S. (2016, August 17). *7 reasons you need a mentor for entrepreneurial success. Entrepreneur*. https://www.entrepreneur.com/article/280134

Eyring, A. (2017, November 8). 4 ways fast-growing companies develop talent for free. *Inc.*. https://www.inc.com/alison-eyring/4-ways-fast-growing-companies-develop-talent-for-free.html

Francis, K.A. (n.d.). The importance of funding for business. *Houston Chronicle*. https://smallbusiness.chron.com/importance-funding-business-59.html

Gatty, A. (n.d.). The benefits of community engagement for your business. *All Business*. https://www.allbusiness.com/the-benefits-of-community-engagement-for-your-business-16768-1.html

Gerber, S. (2014, February 11). 12 ways to foster a more entrepreneurial culture. *Business*. https://www.business.com/articles/12-ways-foster-entrepreneurial-culture/

Gines, D. (2019). The importance of inclusive entrepreneurship. *State of Main* (Winter, 2019). https://higherlogicdownload.s3.amazonaws.com/NMSC/390e0055-2395-4d3b-af60-81b53974430d/UploadedImages/State_of_Main/The_Importance_of_Inclusive_Entrepreneurship_Ecosystems.pdf

Global entrepreneurship index (2018). Global Entrepreneurship and Development Institute. https://thegedi.org/global-entrepreneurship-and-development-index/

Global innovation index 2018. (2018, July 10). World Intellectual Property Association. https://www.wipo.int/pressroom/en/articles/2018/article_0005.html

Goodwin, G. (n.d.). *Confidence by Gabby Goodwin*. https://gabbybows.com/

Heathfield, S. M. (2019, December 29). *Why talent management is an important business strategy to develop*. The Balance Careers. https://www.thebalancecareers.com/what-is-talent-management-really-1919221

Hewlett, S.A., Marshall, M. & Sherbin, L. (2013, December). How diversity can drive innovation. *Harvard Business Review*. https://hbr.org/2013/12/how-diversity-can-drive-innovation

Hodel, K.P. & Meyers, M.E. (2017). *Beyond collisions: how to build entrepreneurial infrastructure*. Wavesource LLC.

Howard, S.G. (2018, January 25). How to build an entrepreneurial culture: 5 tips from Eric Ries. *Fast Company*. https://www.fastcompany.com/90158100/how-to-build-an-entrepreneurial-culture-5-tips-from-eric-ries

Isenber, D. (2011, May 25). Introducing the entrepreneurship ecosystem: Four defining characteristics. *Forbes*. https://www.forbes.com/sites/danisenberg/2011/05/25/introducing-the-entrepreneurship-ecosystem-four-defining-characteristics/#6b4e127d5fe8

Kauffman Foundation. (2018). *Entrepreneurial ecosystem building playbook 3.0*. ESHIP Summit. https://www.kauffman.org/entrepreneurial-ecosystem-building-playbook-draft-2/introduction#aletterfromvictorhwang

Lauckner, S. (2020, July 27). *How many small businesses are in the U.S.? (and other employment stats)*. Fundera. https://www.fundera.com/blog/small-business-employment-and-growth-statistics

McMahon, E.T. (2019). A proven economic development strategy. *State of Main.* https://higherlogicdownload.s3.amazonaws.com/NMSC/UploadedImages/13ab8d07-fa39-46c8-a581-c8fc135fdb81/A_Proven_Economic_Development_Strategy.pdf

Malecki, E.J. (2018, January 8). Entrepreneurship and entrepreneurial ecosystems. John Wiley & Sons. https://doi.org/10.1111/gec3.12359

Merkovich, A. (2019, March 25). 15 entrepreneurship statistics you should know. *Fit Small Business.* https://fitsmallbusiness.com/entrepreneurship-statistics/

Miller, J. (2013, December 9). Science says art will make your kids better thinkers (and nicer people). *Fast Company.* https://www.fastcompany.com/3023094/science-says-art-will-make-your-kids-better-thinkers-and-nicer-people

MyCorporation. (2018, August 8). What is seed money and how can entrepreneurs get it? *StartupNation.* https://startupnation.com/start-your-business/seed-money-entrepreneurs-get/

National Science Foundation. (2018, January 24). Report shows United States leads in science and technology as China rapidly advances. *ScienceDaily.* www.sciencedaily.com/releases/2018/01/180124113951.htm

Nayak, S. & Farrington, K. (n.d.). Impact hiring: *A double bottom-line solution to today's entry-level talent needs.* Society of Human Resources Management. https://www.shrm.org/hr-today/trends-and-forecasting/special-reports-and-expert-views/pages/impact-hiring_a_double_bottom-line_solution.aspx

Networking. (n.d.). *Entrepreneur Small Business Encyclopedia.* https://www.entrepreneur.com/encyclopedia/networking

Non-dilutive: Everything you need to know. (2020, July 2). *UpCounsel.* https://www.upcounsel.com/non-dilutive

Olenski, S. (2015, July 20). 8 key tactics for developing employees. *Forbes.* https://www.forbes.com/sites/steveolenski/2015/07/20/8-key-tactics-for-developing-employees/#72eb1286373d

Oracles, The. (2017, August 24). 8 proven networking strategies of successful entrepreneurs. *Success.* https://www.success.com/8-proven-networking-strategies-of-successful-entrepreneurs/

Overton, S. (n.d.). WisePocket products. https://wisepocketproducts.com/

Paying yourself: from startup and beyond (n.d.). *Entrepreneur*. https://www.entrepreneur.com/article/80024

Quednau, R. (2016, April 20). How to encourage entrepreneurship in your town. *Strong Towns*. https://www.strongtowns.org/journal/2016/4/19/how-to-encourage-entrepreneurship-in-your-town

Rittscher, S. (2012, May 31). Six keys to successful networking for entrepreneurs. *Forbes*. https://www.forbes.com/sites/susanrittscher/2012/05/31/six-keys-to-successful-networking-for-entrepreneurs/#580aefa1580b

Russ, S. (2018, May 9). Help your children play out a story and watch them become more creative. *The Conversation*. https://theconversation.com/help-your-children-play-out-a-story-and-watch-them-become-more-creative-61194

Sappin, E. (2016, October 20). 7 ways entrepreneurs drive economic development. *Entrepreneur*. https://www.entrepreneur.com/article/283616

Schmid, G. (2020, July 24). *Small business statistics: 19 essential numbers to know*. Fundera. https://www.fundera.com/blog/small-business-statistics

Siu, E. (2016, December 27). Pay yourself: Why founders should set aside profits every month. *Entrepreneur*. https://www.entrepreneur.com/article/287001

Small business profile. (2018). Office of Advocacy, U.S. Small Business Administration. https://www.sba.gov/sites/default/files/advocacy/2018-Small-Business-Profiles-US.pdf

Social TrendSpotter. (2016, October 20). 4 elements of entrepreneurial culture and how to incorporate them into the social sector. *Medium*. https://medium.com/@socialtrendspot/4-elements-of-entrepreneurial-culture-and-how-to-incorporate-them-into-the-social-sector-b4baee7e3be1

Stam, E. & Spigel, B. (2016, November). *Entrepreneurial ecosystems*. Utrecht University School of Economics. https://www.uu.nl/sites/default/files/rebo_use_dp_2016_1613.pdf

Supporting entrepreneurship. (2011, April 27). University of Wisconsin Extension in cooperation with The Ohio State University Extension and University of Minnesota Extension.

Vaze, S. (2020, April 17). Why diversity is necessary for innovation at the workplace. *Entrepreneur*. https://www.entrepreneur.com/article/349419

Waugh, A. & Miller, J. (n.d.). What is business engagement? *ExploreVR*. https://www.explorevr.org/sites/explorevr.org/files/files/What%20is%20Business%20Engagement.pdf

What is community engagement? (n.d.). Penn State Department of Agricultural Economics, Sociology, and Education. https://aese.psu.edu/research/centers/cecd/engagement-toolbox/engagement/what-is-community-engagement

Wither, D. (2020). 6 ways to improve your entrepreneur network. *Startup Grind*. https://www.startupgrind.com/blog/6-ways-to-improve-your-entrepreneur-network-2/

Young Entrepreneur Council. (2018, June 26). Entrepreneurial networking: 10 approaches you can use. *Forbes*. https://www.forbes.com/sites/theyec/2018/06/26/entrepreneurial-networking-10-approaches-you-can-use/#6a0ae8afe428

Zwilling, M. (2016, August 31). Smart entrepreneurs build startups without investors. *Forbes*. https://www.forbes.com/sites/martinzwilling/2016/08/31/smart-entrepreneurs-build-startups-without-investors/#15376b1041ba

Zwilling, M. (2017, May 25). 7 elements of company culture that ensure your business keeps improving. *Entrepreneur*. https://www.entrepreneur.com/article/293677

Business Attraction and Site Selection

Robert H. Pittman, PhD, PCED

Location factors are essential to attracting, retaining, and expanding businesses, but what do companies look for in the site selection process? Learn about the top site selection factors and discover the opportunities to enhance or build on these factors for your community.

Learning Outcomes

- Participants will review the site selection process.

- Participants will discuss how communities and developers can make their sites and buildings competitive.

- Participants will learn the importance of effective communication between the community developer and the company and/or site selection consultant during the process.

Local businesses are the lifeblood of a community's economy. They provide jobs and incomes for local residents to support themselves and their dependents, and they support the provision of public services through property and other business taxes. With income from their jobs a company's employees also support local services through the taxes they pay on their homes and other property and goods they purchase. Studies have shown that businesses generally contribute more to local government revenues than they consume in government services. Households, on the other hand, often consume more in local services such as public education than they contribute in taxes.

Just as a rising tide lifts all boats, a strong local business sector and economy help build a better community and quality of life for residents in many ways, including well-funded schools, better roads and infrastructure, and more retail shops and restaurants. Should anyone doubt that local businesses help sustain prosperous communities, they should consider the countless unfortunate examples of community devastation from large employer shutdowns. Local businesses come in a variety of shapes and sizes, from large national or international companies to local "mom and pop" stores. However, they all provide local jobs and help support the community.

Local economic development involves a number of policies and strategies but almost always includes recruiting new businesses, helping retain and expand existing businesses, and supporting entrepreneurial activity and new business startups. Success in economic development, however, is highly dependent on success in community development. A good community makes it easier to accomplish all three of these core economic development functions. Obviously, businesses prefer communities with a better workforce, infrastructure, and other critical operating factors, but they also naturally prefer communities with a good overall quality of life. Therefore, community development and economic development are inextricably linked: A better community contributes to successful economic development, and in turn, a stronger local business sector and economy support community development.

Why Do Community and Economic Developers Need to Understand the Business Location Process?

Establishing that community development and economic development are linked still begs the question: How does a community, region, or state succeed in economic development? Many books have been written on this topic, and many more will be written in the future. While this overarching question is well beyond the scope of this chapter, we can address here a key element of economic development success for many localities—the recruitment of new businesses and investment into the community.

Most business location or "site selection" projects involve the comparison of multiple communities and sites to find the best (usually meaning the most profitable) place to build or acquire a new facility. Communities, therefore, are usually in competition with other communities to attract the investment. In fact, winning a site selection project is much like selling any product or service—you must convince the customer that you have the best offer and solution to their needs. Any good salesperson knows that a key to accomplishing this is to understand the customer's needs and decision process. That, in a nutshell, is why community and economic developers should understand the business location and site selection process. In short, know your customer—in this case the company you are trying to attract to your community. These principles also apply to the retention and expansion of existing local businesses, another key element of successful economic development.

It should be noted that this chapter addresses the business location and investment process for goods- and service-producing companies or organizations. This includes companies that manufacture or distribute physical goods or other tangible products, such as software, and companies that offer services such as technical support, consulting, and professional services to a broad geographic market. In the U.S. economy, the service-producing sector is larger than the manufacturing sector. This chapter does not address the location process of local retail outlets, restaurants, or the like, although many of the principles in this chapter apply to the retail sector.

What Motivates the Business Location Process?

Businesses make capital investments in new facilities and equipment for a variety of reasons. While firm size and type of product or service can make a difference in the location decision, the principles are usually very similar. Some common reasons that companies invest in new or expanded facilities include the following.

Growth of existing product or service: Some facility investments are made by firms to increase their production, distribution, support, or warehousing capacity for an existing product. For example, Apple and other smartphone companies have expanded their production capacity as the demand for these products increased rapidly over the past few years. They also increased distribution and customer service capacity to support these products. Firms producing services as opposed to goods face the same challenges. For example, increased demand for virtual meetings and remote work has required companies such as Zoom Video Communications, Inc. to rapidly increase its product development and customer support capacity.

Introduction of new product or service: When a company develops a new product or service, they often require additional capacity. As with the growth of an existing product or service, the first decision a company introducing a new product faces is whether to expand capacity in their current location(s) by reconfiguring their operations and adding on to existing facilities—or build new facilities in other locations. Tesla, Inc. provides an example. While electric cars have been available for many years, several new models have been introduced in recent years as their popularity has increased. Rather than expand its Fremont, California assembly operations, Tesla, Inc. selected Austin, Texas as the site for a new 2,100-

acre auto assembly plant with a capital investment of $1.1 billion employing over 5,000 workers. The plant will build the company's new Cybertruck.

Need to relocate: Sometimes firms make the decision to relocate existing operations. Abandoning an existing facility and moving to another location across town or to another state or country is a very expensive and disruptive process, but in some cases this can be the right business decision. Reasons for this decision can be "push" or "pull" factors or a combination thereof. Unfortunately for the communities where they are currently located, some businesses choose to move because of a poor business climate (*push*). This term encompasses a number of factors such as local taxes, permitting requirements, and the general support or lack thereof that communities provide for their companies. Other businesses may relocate because they believe they can operate more profitably in other communities (*pull*). For example, a firm producing high-technology products may choose to relocate to a community with a college offering a top-notch engineering program.

Obsolescence of existing facilities: Often company facilities can become less productive over time as technologies, product mixes, or both change. For example, new production technologies may require higher ceiling heights or different layouts, rendering an existing single-story facility obsolete. When something like this occurs, a company must make a decision to acquire a new facility where they are currently located or choose a different community. This is where an economic development organization can help save local jobs by working with the company to encourage and support a decision to stay in the community.

Quality of life for owners and executives: While most business location decisions are based on sound economics, not all of them are made solely with spreadsheets. Business owners and key decision-making executives can decide to locate for personal reasons. Years ago, a large firm relocated from upstate New York to Florida. The owner and CEO cited Florida's good business climate—but he was an avid sailboat sportsman so perhaps that was not the only climate he was considering. A good quality of life can also help a firm recruit the best employees, giving it an advantage over competing firms.

Logistical factors: Sometimes a company's customers and markets can shift geographically. Especially for firms whose raw materials and products involve significant transportation costs—or who have the need to minimize delivery time to customers—it may become prudent to locate or expand in a different area to align with those shifts. Several years ago, California-based Dole, Inc. built a second plant in Ohio to produce packaged salads to better serve a growing demand in the eastern U.S. It made economic sense for the company to move production closer to their customers instead of shipping a perishable product across the country.

Amazon HQ2

One of the most publicized company expansions in recent years was the location decision for Amazon's second headquarters, or HQ2. More than 200 locations submitted proposals to win the project and its thousands of high-paying jobs. From those initial candidates, 20 finalists were selected for further evaluation. Each site was visited by Amazon executives during which local officials made their pitches. In November 2018 Amazon announced that it would split its new headquarters facilities between two locations, New York City (specifically Long Island City) and northern Virginia. To win such as plum project, virtually all the initial bidders offered incentives such as tax abatements and workforce training, and these initial offers were refined in negotiations with the finalist cities. As it turned out, the incentive race reversed the Long Island City location decision because of local opposition to corporate "give-aways" and the impact that the company's operations would have on local neighborhoods. According to Amazon, the project includes a $5 billion construction budget and will ultimately create 50,000 jobs, offering huge economic benefits to the winning location(s). This project is a reminder that new white-collar or office facilities can have as much or more of an impact on a local economy as production facilities.

Who Are the Decision Makers?

Larger companies serving global markets regularly make facility location and expansion decisions because of the number and variety of their products. Executives in these companies are often more experienced and comfortable with the process and usually have corporate support staff to assist such as human resource departments to evaluate the local workforce in candidate locations. Depending on the size and organization of the company and magnitude of the investment, the location decision can be made by the particular division or department involved in the expansion or at a higher corporate management level. Below are some of the common final decision makers for a facility location:

- **The CEO or president** sometimes takes it upon him/herself to make the final decision. This is more likely to be the case in smaller closely held companies.

- Some location decisions are made by a **division or department** within a company for which a new facility is needed. The managing executives and operations specialists within a division are most knowledgeable about their particular product or service and therefore are often the most qualified to find the best community and site for a new facility. On the other hand, when location decisions involve operations that cut across divisions, such as corporate or regional headquarters facilities, they are usually made by top "C suite" corporate executives.

- A **committee or special team** with division executives and corporate support departments is a very common configuration for making facility investment and location decisions. Such teams usually include a top management representative (e.g., a production manager) from the division for which a new facility is needed, a representative from the corporate real estate department familiar with building or leasing facilities, someone from the human resources department to help evaluate local workforces, and someone from financial operations to help measure the costs and returns from the new facility.

- In some cases, an **individual executive** is assigned to supervise the location decision process. This person would be wise to put together a team as described above to help with all aspects of the location decision rather than try to go it alone.

- For some projects, companies hire **business location consultants** to help make a decision. These consultants have experience in the site selection and community evaluation process that companies can benefit from. The extent of their role in the decision varies. Some consultants are given full rein to manage the location decision process, while others are just given special assignments such as data collection and analysis.

- Industrial and commercial **real estate agents** usually play a role in a corporate expansion, either in purchasing an existing facility or acquiring land to build a new one. While their role is usually limited to facilitating the acquisition of a building or site, some companies assign them larger roles and some national real estate companies have their own in-house site selection consultants.

For smaller companies with one or just a few facilities, the expansion and location decisions tend to be less complex and are normally made by owners or key management executives. Smaller companies typically do not conduct costly and time-consuming site searches across a number of states and localities, often relying instead on local economic development agencies and real estate agents in areas they are familiar with or know they need to expand in. Smaller companies are less likely to engage site selection consultants to help them decide on facility locations.

Except for some larger companies with a variety of products and markets and more rapid growth, facility location decisions are a relatively rare event. Consequently, company representatives making the decision are often less familiar with the site selection process and how to make a good decision than economic developers or other local representatives that often deal with companies looking at their communities. Inexperience can make company location decision makers tentative and uncertain and more risk averse. Selecting a new location and building or acquiring a new facility is not like purchasing a consumer product—you cannot return the product and get a refund after the facility is built and new employees hired. This inexperience can create opportunities for local economic developers and community leaders to be considered more like partners than sales representatives to companies looking for a new location. Treating the company well, satisfying its needs, reducing its perceived risk, and most importantly, solving its problem is the key to winning the project. Knowing who the final decision maker is in any situation is a key to closing the deal.

How the Business Location Process Works

As noted above, there are usually differences in the way larger and smaller companies go about the site selection process. Big companies that produce goods or services on a large scale for broad geographic markets make larger investments and tend to follow a more systematic process. Smaller companies that produce a limited product line are typically not making a large facility investment and do not want to spend the time and money involved in a multistate site search. In addition, often the operations of smaller companies are overseen by an owner or founder, making it difficult to manage distant facilities. To distinguish these two types of site searches, we will call them *systematic* and *ad hoc*.

The Systematic Approach

When a larger company decides that it needs to increase capacity for any of the reasons discussed above, it first goes through a facility and location needs assessment. This can be divided up into three parts:

- Physical facility and site needs
- Geographic location requirements
- Local market requirements

Physical Facility and Site Needs

The first issue to be addressed is obviously what will be produced in the new facility, followed by the physical requirements of the site and building to efficiently produce those goods or services. How large should the building be, and how should it be laid out (ceiling height, mix of production vs. office space, etc.)? What are the physical site requirements (parking, ingress/egress, etc.)? There is also the question of future capacity requirements—how will the production space requirements change in the future as product sales grow? Should the company go ahead and provide space for future growth when they acquire or build a facility—or wait and see what the future brings? A compromise strategy might be to acquire only the space needed for immediate operations but provide flexibility by purchasing a larger site that could accommodate future expansion. For a company looking only for new office space, the physical facility criteria are obviously somewhat different, but the process is the same. Facility planning is a complex undertaking involving architects, engineers, and company management and operations personnel—and a whole topic unto itself.

Geographic Location Requirements

In addition to specifying the physical site and building needs, a company must determine the broad geographical location requirements. Where in the country or world should the new facility be located? Some common questions entering into this decision include:

- **Is the facility tied to certain inputs that are location-specific?** This can be the case, for example, when a mined product is a key input to production.

- **Is the facility tied to certain geographic product markets?** Is there a need for the product or service to be produced in close proximity to its consumers?

- **What is the best logistical location?** This factor often involves both of the above two questions. Where are the locations that provide cost- and time-efficient assembly of production inputs and shipment of finished product? This is particularly important for distribution facilities for companies such as Amazon and Wayfair that offer fast home delivery. Auto assembly plants rely on thousands of parts from many different suppliers, and all involved in this supply chain must take that interconnectedness into account when deciding on a location.

- **How will the new facility geographically fit in with the company's existing facilities?** Production of a particular product is often spread among many company locations. Intermediate products, or goods in progress, are often shipped to another company location for final production.

- **Are there public relations or corporate marketing considerations?** Some companies want their locations to make a statement or serve to enhance their image. For example, auto assembly plants are almost always located on interstate highways. Transportation of inputs and outputs (finished automobiles) is an important driver of this location preference, but visibility and convenience for visitors are also commonly considered by the auto companies.

Local Market Requirements

Geographic location requirements can influence the site selection decision to varying degrees. In the case of warehouses to serve home delivery companies like Amazon or provide inventory for stores like Walmart, the logistics are often the overriding concern and point to a specific location. However, for many companies, the geographical location requirements are less strict and can be met by locating in a particular section of the country such as, for example, the Southeast or a few contiguous states elsewhere. Once the general geographic location is determined, a specific community and site within the area must be found, and many local market factors must be considered. The accompanying box lists some of the factors that are commonly considered when deciding which community and site—and broader geographic area—to select.

Common Country and Regional Location Factors

- Product markets
- Raw material location sources
- Transportation networks
- Competitor locations
- Location of existing facilities
- Energy cost and policies
- Labor (cost, availability, regulations, and policies)
- Business climate (taxes, regulations, attitudes towards businesses, etc.)

Some Common State Location Factors

- Business taxes
- Personal taxes
- Workers' compensation laws and rates
- Unemployment insurance laws and rates
- Right-to-work legislation (right to not join a union)
- Incentives
- General business climate (receptivity and attitude toward businesses)

Some Common Community Location Factors

- Availability of sites and/or buildings meeting project needs
- Local transportation (roads, access to major highways, public transportation, etc.)
- Nonlocal transportation (air service, highways, rail service, etc.)
- Labor (availability, productivity and work ethic, cost)
- Labor relations
- Education (K–12, post-secondary, technical schools)
- Training (state or local sponsored programs, technical degree programs)
- Utilities (service, quality, cost)
- Quality of life
- Size and growth of community
- Incentives
- Environmental policies

The Request for Proposals

Once the larger geographic search area is determined, the task remains to choose from among the hundreds of potential locations within that broader territory. It would be a gargantuan task for a company to gather and review information on all of these communities and sites. Instead, they normally rely on states, regions, and communities to provide information to them on sites that best meet their criteria. This is most easily done through issuing a Request for Proposals (RFP) containing questions and requesting information on the specific needs of a company's expansion project such as those listed on the previous page. The location requirements—and therefore the RFP—are specific, and there are no one-size-fits-all site selection "checklists." RFPs can be long and formal documents (some consultants and companies are famous for this) or short with just a few key questions.

The RFPs are normally distributed to state departments of economic development (or counties) in the general search areas that are familiar with their communities and sites and can select the ones that best meet the location criteria in the RFP. Normally, each state will submit five to ten communities and sites. RFPs are sometimes also sent to larger utility companies with economic development departments that maintain databases of available sites and buildings and other regional and local information relevant to a location decision.

Case Study
Where in the World Do We Expand?

Executives of a company located in the Midwest making medical products once contacted a consultant for help with a challenging expansion question. Their products were selling well throughout the U.S. and had recently caught on in Europe. The U.S. demand could be met by their production facility in the Midwest, but they were having difficulty meeting European demand. As a temporary measure, they had signed a short-term lease for a facility in a major European city to which they could ship partially produced goods for final production and warehouse for distribution. The city was expensive, and their operating costs there were quite high, but they were not familiar with how to find another location in Europe. Another issue they faced was rising demand for their products in Australia. They had been meeting that demand by adding a third shift to their plant in the Midwest.

The company faced many expansion and location unknowns and questions discussed in this chapter. How fast would product demand increase in Europe and Australia? Would it be more efficient to expand U.S. production capacity to meet worldwide demand, or should they add facilities in Europe and Australia to meet demand growth in those areas? Where should they locate their facilities overseas?

After an assessment of their situation, the consultant recommended that production capacity be expanded in their Midwest location to serve worldwide demand. There were many reasons for this recommendation, including:

- challenges to maintaining consistent product quality in multiple production locations;

- higher production costs overseas, especially in Europe;

- uncertainty regarding future medical product regulations in Europe and Australia;

- uncertainty regarding product demand growth and the entry of potential competitors in overseas markets.

The company agreed that the risks of expanding overseas exceeded the potential reward of growing market share through expanding their facilities overseas. They doubled their production space and capacity at their Midwest location, creating almost 100 new jobs for local residents. And, according to one executive, they slept better at night.

Site Selection or Elimination?

Once states and other entities receiving the RFP respond to it with locations in their territory they believe match the requirements in the RFP and will be competitive in the final decision, the process to make the final selection begins. This is typically a three-phase approach as illustrated by the accompanying figure.

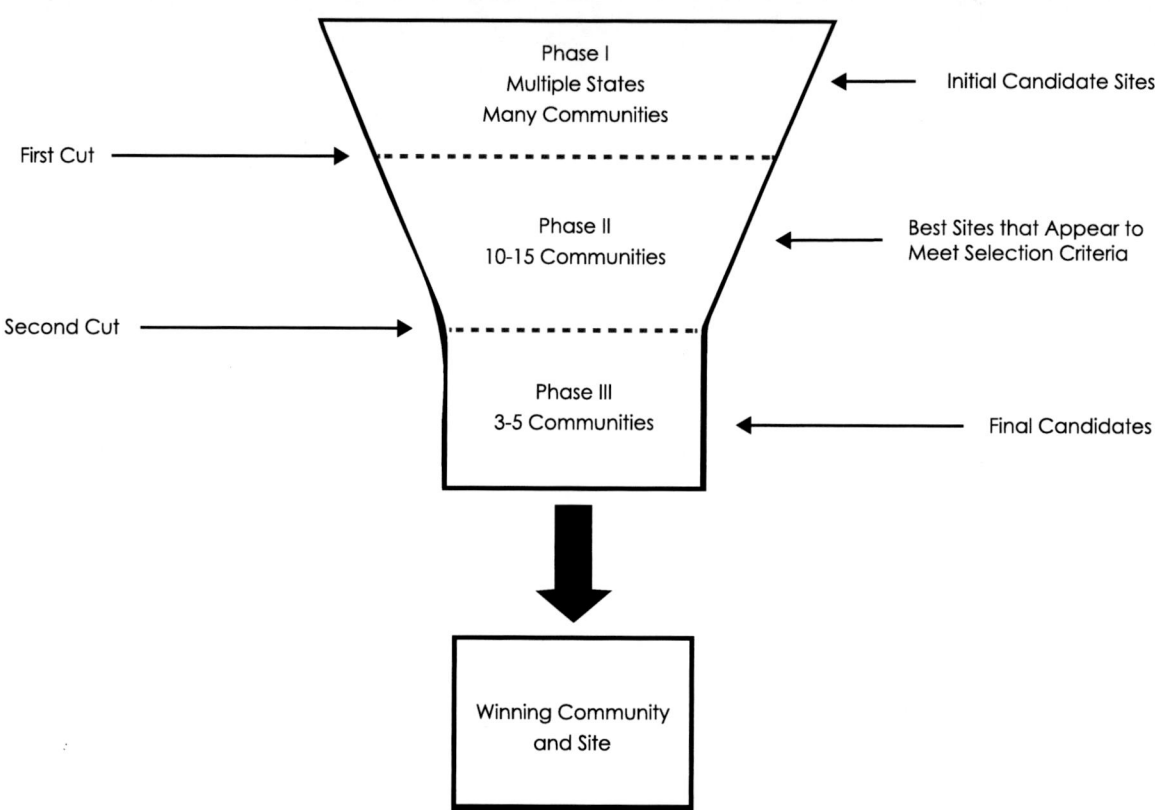

Typical Three-Phase Facility Site Selection Process

Phase I: First cut. If the general search area is large and contains several states or even countries, the number of initial submittals can be large—often 50 to 100 or more—and they can be quite long. One approach would be to read all the proposals cover to cover and then pick the winner, but that would be extremely time-consuming. The more efficient way is to screen the proposals and eliminate those that for one reason or another do not meet the criteria well or not at all. For example, water and sewer service might be very important to a food processing company. Some of the submitted communities might have very little excess water and sewer treatment capacity, and so could be eliminated at the outset for fear that service could be compromised at some future date. Phase I screening typically results in a sorting of the proposals in to three groups: (1) those that appear to meet all location criteria; (2) those that clearly do not; and (3) the "maybe" stack. This is the first cut in the process.

Phase II: Second cut—candidates for further evaluation. Proposals that survive the first cut in Phase I and that appear on paper to meet the location criteria (say 10 to 15, but the numbers vary) then undergo further scrutiny. At this point, the semifinalist locations are generally contacted by the consultant or company with requests for more information or additional questions. The company or consultant typically does additional research and gathers more data on the remaining communities from their websites, independent demographic and economic data vendors, and other sources. Financial modeling to evaluate the profitability of each proposed site is often undertaken at this point. A spreadsheet is created containing rows for various production cost and revenue items such as wage rates, taxes, transportation costs, etc. Subjective factors that cannot be easily measured with a number, such as overall receptivity to new business, can be assigned a qualitative score such as A, B or C. This initial financial modeling helps identify the locations that move on to final consideration. It is also typical for representatives from the company and/or consultant to visit some or all of the Phase II location candidates to inspect the proposed site or building, interview local business owners concerning their experience with the community, and get a feel for the local quality of life.

Phase III: The finalists. The detailed evaluations and site visits for the semifinal candidates in Phase II provide the quantitative and qualitative information to narrow the choice down (the second cut) to the final candidates, from which the best community and site for the project will be chosen. At this point, even more detailed data may be collected or requested, and in-depth discussions are conducted with the finalist communities on any issues of concern. Typically, negotiations on incentives are conducted. Through these negotiations, the proposals for the remaining communities are finalized and the stage is set for the final selection.

Selecting the winner. In some cases, there is a clear winner from among the finalists, and in other cases it can be a hard choice to make. By definition, the remaining locations meet the RFP criteria and Phase II screening, or they wouldn't be a Phase III finalist. At this point the final decision sometimes comes down to subjective factors such as which communities the company executives prefer to live in, or image and perception issues for the company. The relationship and trust the finalist communities have developed with the company and the knowledge of its specific preferences by this point in the process can often help win the project.

Economic Development Incentives

The term *incentives* in the economic development sense refers to certain considerations given to companies by governments to encourage them to locate in their state or locality. Some common types of incentives include:

- tax exemptions or reductions
- job creation credits
- dpecial utility rates
- expedited permitting
- low-interest loans
- reduced price for land and buildings
- infrastructure development and site preparation
- labor training

Incentives can be broadly classified into two groups. The first, *statutory incentives*, refers to incentives that are based on laws already passed and available to any company that qualifies for them. A common example is job tax credits. In an effort to stimulate and reward job creation, several states provide tax credits (a reduction in taxed income or direct reduction in taxes payable) for net new jobs a company creates in that state in a given year. This normally applies both to new companies moving in and companies already located in the state. The second type, *negotiated incentives*, refers to special incentives that are negotiated between a state and locality and a company. They are commonly associated with larger highly visible projects for which many states and localities are competing (see Case Study).

Incentives are sometimes described as "corporate welfare" or "giving away public tax dollars." There are two sides to this argument. As discussed in the introduction to this chapter, companies create jobs, tax revenues, and many other benefits for the communities in which they operate. The rationale for incentives is that they are necessary for states and localities to be viable in the competition to attract business investment. Furthermore, the value of the incentives given to the company is usually much less than the benefits to the state and community and its residents from the company, including increased tax revenues and new jobs and incomes. If this is not the case, then the incentives should be pared back.

Claims that states and communities "lure" companies with incentives are misleading. Incentives such as tax abatements almost always have a time limitation to them—five to ten years is common. In the financial analysis companies conduct to compare different location options (in Phase II in the Site Selection Process diagram) the value of incentives is usually much less important to the bottom line than other cost and revenue factors. There is a saying among site selection consultants: "Incentives do not make a bad site good." States and communities should be wary of a company looking for a site that first asks about incentives. Such companies usually fall into one of two categories: those that are financially weak and need immediate relief, and those that are playing a bargaining game with the governments where they are currently located and seeking the leverage of another incentive offer. Incentives are very often tiebreakers in the Phase III final search process and are just one of many tools to help recruit companies or encourage existing local companies to create more jobs. By themselves, however, incentives cannot be the basis of a successful economic development strategy.

The Ad Hoc Approach

While many larger companies go through something like the Three-Phase approach to finding a site, smaller companies, as previously noted, typically do not have the need or resources for this systematic method. They are often looking for a building or site close to where they are currently located. Executives of these companies can utilize a variety of resources in their search, including industrial and commercial realtors, direct contact with local and regional economic development organizations, or simply word-of-mouth.

This does not imply, however, that communities and economic development organizations should give smaller companies less attention than larger ones. Studies have shown that the expansion of existing small companies and the startup of new businesses typically create more jobs in a community than larger businesses moving into the area. This is true for several reasons, including the fact that recruiting companies from outside the area is very competitive, with dozens or sometimes hundreds of localities trying to win a project. For this and other reasons, an important component of a community's economic development strategy should be programs to help retain and expand local businesses and encourage the creation of new ones.

Keys to Winning Business Investment Projects

As noted elsewhere in this chapter, each business location/site selection project is unique in the specific needs companies have and the exact way they go about finding a suitable community and site. Winning the competition for these projects is a science as well as an art. The science involves practicing good community development, having a good "product" that is attractive to companies, and having the resources to quickly and appropriately respond to RFPs and other location inquiries. The art involves knowing how the business location process works and how to win the competition. Below are some key points or best practices to keep in mind to help attract business investment to a community, region, or state:

- **Know your customer as well as you can.** Why is the company wanting to expand? What are the major requirements the company has for the new building and/or site? Who are the ultimate decision makers in the process? Keep in mind that the process is about meeting the needs of the customer and solving the company's problem, not just relying on a one-size-fits-all promotion for your community.

- **Follow the rules of the game as specified for a particular project.** An RFP for a business location project usually has very specific guidelines for submitting information and participating in the process. Even more informal business location inquiries usually have a specified process. In a three-phase or similar process as outlined in this chapter, the community's goal should be to make it to the next round—through the first cut to the semifinals and through the second cut to the finals. In other words, you must make it to first, second, and then third base before you score a run.

- **Be completely responsive to RFPs and other business location inquiries.** Provide all information in the way it is requested. Never answer a question with a phrase such as "The information you requested is contained in the attached brochure."

- **Be professional, prompt, and user-friendly** throughout the entire process from responding to the RFP to providing additional information as the process moves forward.

- **Understand your community's strengths and weaknesses** and suitability for different kinds of investments and industries. For example, a rural community away from an interstate highway is not going to win a project like an automobile assembly plant. A community should seek to generate more RFPs from state departments of economic development by keeping them and other lead sources informed on the types of investment projects the community is suitable for and desires.

- **Educate key people in your community,** such as elected officials and experts in important subject areas (e.g, utilities, transportation, planning and zoning, workforce training, etc.) on how the business location process works so they will be better prepared to help win the project. This will also help ensure that a community provides the necessary resources to support a good economic development program that can respond to inquiries—and better yet, implement a marketing outreach campaign to generate more inquiries.

- **Be prepared to respond quickly to RFPs** or other requests for information. This means that communities must have the personnel and resources (e.g., reliable, complete, and objective data) to respond (sometimes literally overnight) as requested.

- Location projects are often confidential with code names to prevent any difficulties for the company. **Never violate that confidentiality.**

- **Always remember that any business location project is about the needs of the customer,** not the mayor *(Let me take the lead, I know how!)* or an economic development board member *(I have a 20-acre cornfield, but it could make a nice industrial site, so let's submit it!)*.

These are but a few of the keys to attracting business investment into a community. A good place to start is the subject of this chapter—how business location processes and decisions generally work.

Concluding Observations

Success in community and economic development does not happen by accident. However, the basic formula for success is straightforward: follow the principles of community development to create a place where businesses and individuals want to live and then market it to the desired audiences. In practice, of course, this is not easy to do. Instructions on how to ride a bicycle can also seem straightforward: sit on the seat, put your feet on the pedals, push off, and pedal. But in practice, riding a bicycle involves balance, knowing the rules of the road, and many other factors that must be mastered. The practice of community and economic development, like learning to ride a bicycle, is harder than the theory.

Community development and economic development go hand in hand. This chapter has demonstrated this symbiotic link from yet another perspective—that of attracting business investment into a community. A key factor for success is understanding the business location process.

Case Study
Understanding and Solving the Client's Problem

This was a plum of a project—one that many states and communities competed for because, well, you just had to go for this one. An aerospace company was looking for a location to design and build a new product for use in space exploration. This was a high-dollar project all around with hundreds of millions of dollars in investment and hundreds of jobs for high-paid engineers and other employees. The economic impact—from construction jobs, permanent jobs, taxes, and other direct benefits—would be huge for the chosen community and state. But the indirect benefits promised to be just as large. The highly paid employees would buy houses and pay residential property taxes, shop local stores, and put money in the pockets of local merchants and sales tax revenues in state and local coffers. In addition, winning a project like this would enhance the prestige of the chosen community and state and demonstrate they were competitive for world-class projects.

Obviously not all communities would be suitable for a project of this magnitude. A larger community would be necessary to supply a workforce, housing, local infrastructure, public services, and other needs for a project of this magnitude. For the company to attract and retain the highly skilled labor force, the location would need to offer a high quality of life. Furthermore, there was a political angle to this decision. Elected officials at the local, state, and national levels would be lobbying this aerospace company to locate in their jurisdictions, and some of these officials would have some influence over government purchases of the company's products. All in all, this was an important project for the company and the competing communities, and the final decision had to be carefully made and justified.

With the help of a consultant, the company drew up a Request for Proposals (RFP) containing a detailed list of "needs" (must haves) and "wants" (would be nice, but not absolutely necessary). The list covered a broad array of location-decision factors including labor (availability, skill levels, cost), suitable sites, infrastructure, and utilities—with a special emphasis on K–12 and higher education resources because of the high-tech nature of the product. Detailed information on state and local taxes was also requested.

While some states knew they would not be competitive in the selection process because of location, transportation, small markets, and other factors (e.g., Alaska, Hawaii, and some other smaller population states), many states did answer the RFP, proposing several of their communities and sites that they thought would make a good match for the project. In the usual manner of making location decisions described in this chapter, the consultant and company reviewed the proposals, eliminating some at this first stage because they did not meet or poorly met the RFP criteria. Surviving this first cut were about 15 communities and sites that appeared to adequately meet the selection criteria, but that bore further study and for some, a visit.

After this second round, three states—with a specific site in each one—remained in contention. As described in this chapter, the "tie-breaking" or final selection process then began. Representatives from each of the three states and the community they proposed met with the company in the consultant's office to make their final pitches, answer questions, and negotiate a final package offer, including incentives. At this down-to-the-brass-tacks point, the company confided that they needed some relief from each state's inventory tax on goods-in-progress because their aerospace product was hugely expensive and took months to produce. Because of this, the inventory tax, really designed for products of more nominal value that were more quickly produced, would be prohibitive. Here is how the states responded to that request:

- State A: "Our legal counsel informs us that inventory tax relief would be very difficult to do and would set a bad precedent for us. We're sorry, what else can we do for you?"

- State B: "Our legislature is not in session for another three months, but at that time we promise to introduce legislation to give you some inventory tax relief."

- State C: "Give us a week to address this issue, and please don't make a decision until then." The next week, the governor of State C called the legislature into special session and passed an inventory tax relief bill for companies producing such big-ticket, high-tech products.

A multiple choice test: Who won the project? Of course the answer is C. That state immediately solved the problem and indicated a willingness to work with the company to make it successful. State A was immediately eliminated from the competition. State B might have solved the problem, but it would take at least three months and the legislative outcome was uncertain, introducing delay and risk into the company's project. The cost of the inventory tax reduction and other incentives was dwarfed by the huge economic impact to the state and chosen community. All three states knew that, but State C was able to immediately address one of the company's most pressing needs in the final selection round.

This case study illustrates a key point in this chapter: states and communities that understand the needs of their business "clients" (businesses already located there and new businesses looking for a location) and act quickly and decisively to address them can put themselves a step ahead of the competition and win projects.

References

Gerdeman, D. (2012). Location, Location, Location: The Strategy of Place. *Working Knowledge*.

Jensen, N. M., Malesky, E. J., & Walsh, M. (2015). Competing for global capital or local voters? The politics of business location incentives. *Springer Link*. https://link.springer.com/article/10.1007/s11127-015-0281-8

Kimelberg, S. M., & Williams, E. (2013). Evaluating the Importance of Business Location Factors: The Influence of Facility Type. *Growth and Change*. https://onlinelibrary.wiley.com/doi/abs/10.1111/grow.12003

Phillips, R., & Pittman, R. (2014). *An Introduction to Community Development, 2nd Edition*. Routledge.

Pittman, R. H. (2006). Location, Location, Location: Winning Site Selection Proposals. *Management Quarterly*.

Pittman, R., Pittman, E., & Phillips, R. (2009). The Community and Economic Development Chain: Validating the Links Between Processes and Outcomes. *ResearchGate*. https://www.researchgate.net/publication/233242539_The_Community_and_Economic_Development_Chain_Validating_the_Links_Between_Processes_and_Outcomes

Various. (n.d.). Retrieved from Prosperous Places: https://www.prosperousplaces.org/

Various. (n.d.). Site Selection Magazine. *Site Selection Magazine*. Retrieved from https://siteselection.com/#gsc.tab=0

Business Retention and Expansion

Dennis E. Williamson II, PCED, BREC

This course covers the basic components of a successful business retention and expansion (BRE) program and why nurturing and supporting existing businesses is so critical to a community's economic health. Participants will also learn how to increase the competitiveness of local businesses as well as job creation strategies and cost-effective approaches to economic development, including the role individual community members can play in supporting a BRE program.

Learning Outcomes

- Participants will review the three-legged stool of economic development: recruitment, small business development/entrepreneurship, and business retention and expansion.

- Participants will study the rationale for, and history of, BRE.

- Participants will learn about BRE programs (incentives, training, visitation programs, executives' roundtable, etc.) and barriers to BRE.

According to the U.S. Small Business Administration's Office of Advocacy *Small Business Profile* for 2019, 99.9% of all businesses in the United States are considered small businesses and represent 47.3% of jobs in the United States (*Small Business Profile*, 2019). All businesses in our communities are important, but who will advocate and assist those with the fewest resources? How can your community mobilize to be inclusive and partner with all businesses, large and small? If we want to encourage growth, diversity, innovation, and inclusivity in our communities it is important that we connect with the entities that are the base of local economies and truly make them a part of our communities' fabric.

In this chapter you will be exposed to local advocacy through the program concept called Business Retention and Expansion (BRE). We will look at tools of this growth strategy, review steps to developing a program, and discuss how it connects to economic development. We hope to encourage you to review resources available locally to determine an approach that can work for your community. We will look at aspects of various BRE programs to understand the connection to economic development and learn about resources outside our communities that may have value to you.

What is Business Retention and Expansion?

In economic development, business retention and expansion is a program designed to strengthen the connection between companies and the community while encouraging each business to continue to grow. Through direct interactions, events, and research, the program seeks to gain insight into business practices, planned future actions, and the challenges of targeted companies. Practitioners then work in partnership to turn this "business intelligence" into value-added services, programs, and/or products that address individual and shared company opportunities and problems ("What is BR&E?," 2018). BRE has been practiced for decades. The execution and outcomes have changed over time. In the 1960s and '70s the objective was to provide an informal relationship-building tool between businesses and the community. It has progressed to focus more on providing tools and services that assist local firms in competitiveness and growth where they are rather than relocate. This proves to be a more cost-efficient means of developing local jobs and revenue than attracting new businesses (Farnsworth, Clark, & Cochran, n.d.).

To illustrate this, let us explore the concept of the three-legged stool that supports economic development. The theory is that recruitment, startup or creation, and business retention and expansion are the three legs that support economic development. Startup and new business creation carries high risk and typically takes time to produce quality sustainable results, as evidenced by the failure rates illustrated in an article quoting the Bureau of Labor Statistics that 65% of new businesses do not make it beyond 10 years (Deane, 2020). Recruitment is the most highly publicized element of economic development. It is glamorous, often nets large infusions of capital investment and sometimes brings new jobs to a community selected to be the home site. However, recruitment is usually costly and the process lengthy; the community's commitments can be substantial provided the community is even suitable as a host site. In brief, recruitment of a new company to your community can take a long period to provide a positive return on investment.

This brings us to the business retention and expansion approach of economic development. This avenue is often overlooked, since the businesses already operate in our communities, providing jobs and revenue to the local area. They are run by neighbors and friends, which may be why we do not think to appreciate what the company provides or ask if these companies are having any challenges. It is often overlooked that local businesses may have needs to grow. They might have issues they do not know how to overcome and need information on available resources to offset challenges to that growth and existence in our towns.

Why Business Retention and Expansion?

What is easier—to create something new or maintain and improve something we are already familiar with? The cost and resources needed to keep a business in your community will typically be lower than trying to attract something new. You know your local businesses and many of the people who run them, so there is already a connection to the community. We use and depend on them daily, whether it is the services they provide, products we consume, or simply the jobs and revenue they produce. Do you thank them for being there, for the service they provide, for the revenues generated that pay for other services our communities rely on? We often overlook sharing our appreciation to the businesses that already exist, taking for granted that they know the community cares. The old adage is you don't know what you have until it is gone. Recognition and acknowledgment are an important output of the program. After all, you want them to stay around.

A BRE program can help strengthen ties between local businesses and community stakeholders and entice them to become more involved. A quality and well promoted program can also send a message that your community is business-friendly and inclusive; this can move you up the radar for companies that may be looking for a new location and invigorate an entrepreneurial spirit in local residents (Teamwork Arkansas, 2005, p. 10).

A BRE program can provide a structured and methodical means to understand what is going on with the businesses in your community. If approached with purpose it can be designed to meet short-, medium-, and long-term goals for growth in a community. Whether your community is tourist-focused, a bedroom community, reliant on manufacturing or any of dozens of other industry sectors a well-planned BRE program is vital to the overall health of the local area. Your citizens rely on these businesses for employment, services, or shopping needs; to overlook what you have can have catastrophic consequences.

So, the point of creating and executing business retention and expansion is to understand the businesses in your area. To know who they really are and what makes them run, it is important to make sure they are connected to the community and not just left to fend for themselves until they give up or find a more inviting location. By communicating with businesses, you can also make sure they have what they need to prosper and grow.

Variations of Business Retention and Expansion Programs

Business retention and expansion programs are as varied as the number of practitioners who develop and manage them. Many practitioners will put their own spin on the project based upon the resources and team members they can recruit to the cause. Programs may be developed to focus on a specific city or area within a city. They may be built on a regional concept designed around related sectors or warranted by negative impacts within the area. It may also be necessitated due to limited resources or the spread of businesses over an area, especially when the area is more rural. Programs may be designed to focus on particular industry sectors or based upon those most vulnerable. During the current pandemic, programs have been developed to understand the job market—from the perspective of both the company and jobseekers—to determine how to align resources to provide as holistic a solution menu as possible in preparing for the uncertainty of future need.

Two models most recognized that we will discuss here are the *traditional model* that utilizes volunteers and the *continuous model* operated by a permanent paid staff (Jacobs, 2016, p. 7). Program design may use a dedicated paid staff, volunteers, or some combination of the two. A paid program or continuous model will typically consist of a small number of specialized staff to execute the various components of the project. This type of program is designed to operate continuously, year after year. Resources will determine the number of paid staff and may consist of a director, marketer, visitation specialist, solutions specialist, and support staff. With a dedicated staff, the program makes regular business contacts, setting appointments for visitation staff who gather information to be processed by a solutions team who will follow up regarding identified issues or questions. This type of program typically has some form of funding in place to ensure that the BRE activities continue year to year. One example of a funded program with permanent paid staff is BusinessFirst! in the Dayton, Ohio, region, which helps the organization present a single point of contact for a large geographic area with consistent business contact year-round.

On the other hand, an area with limited resources will likely rely heavily on a team of volunteers to provide the various segments of program application. This is the traditional model typically made up of a coalition of organizations or individuals who carry out the program. Membership often utilizes a chamber of commerce or its leadership, employees of the city or municipality, local leaders, economic and workforce development staff, and businesspeople. An example of this is the city of Van Buren, Arkansas, working in cooperation with the Western Arkansas Planning and Development District and relying on community business leaders, the mayor, district staff, and chamber of commerce staff, all of whom volunteer to perform program tasks outside their normal job duties. Community buy-in can have a significant impact on the makeup of the program group. Note that it is still essential to follow a similar protocol of leadership, contact, visitation, data review, and solution resolution to create a successful project. With a volunteer program it is important to qualify individual team members to the task assigned. All it takes is one bad encounter, and the project could be maligned with the area businesses and even the community at large.

The number of businesses a BRE program can reach in a given period of time needs to be determined. This will be affected by the number of people and resources dedicated to the business retention and expansion program. These same factors will have a bearing on how quickly solutions and resolution may be provided as well as regular follow-up. No matter the approach, a response of some kind needs to be presented to the business in a reasonable amount of time after visiting. Remember, the business retention and expansion teams have one goal, and that is to promote community and business relationships, not sell another program or—the worst-case scenario—divulge trade secrets or competitive advantages.

The Visitation Process

Visitation in a business retention and expansion program is a structured and continuous process. The goal is to accomplish a couple of things: acknowledge the importance of the business to the community (usually in the form of a simple thank-you) and give the company representative the opportunity to explain what they do. The visitation team can guide the conversation: What pain points are they facing? How involved are they with the community? What are their goals for the future? Most business owners welcome the chance to brag and address questions about the state of activity for the business,

Whether the program is being executed by a paid staff or volunteers, it is key to provide training on what a visitation should consist of, how to perform a visitation, and the questions to be covered as a conversation (rather than just checking boxes on a list). Visitation staff should be comfortable creating an interactive session to get the most out of the visit and to build a rapport with key representatives of the business. After all, you do want to be welcomed back and need quality communications to provide a growth environment for these key elements that promote a healthy community.

An important component of a successful business retention and expansion program is confidentiality. Business is difficult enough; if a business owner fears a person may divulge trade secrets that set them apart that can be hard to overcome. My advice is to address this in your planning and make your stance on confidentiality obvious so you can get the critical information you need to help businesses in your community. This can also go a long way in building rapport with business and industry and ensuring greater buy-in to the BRE program.

Another important aspect of the visitation process is to create a platform or series of questions and conversation that will provide a consistent data set of feedback. This is relevant to the process in that you are trying to establish clear understanding of what the BRE program can produce and identifying common factors that may be affecting businesses in the program area. It is also necessary to evaluate the questions asked and the time it will take to perform a quality visit. Time is money, and business professionals are always short on time.

One type of visitation, the *business walk*, is a simple and informal way to cover a lot of ground in a designated period of time. This form of outreach is used by many developer organizations.

The BusinessFirst! programs of the greater Dayton region in Ohio and the city of Quesnel in British Columbia, Canada have active Business Walk programs. They are independent programs from different parts of the world executing similar outreach. Chambers of commerce have been using this type of visitation for a long time. A small team made up of BRE program members, community leaders, local chamber staff, and local officials canvasses a designated business area, informally meeting with businesses and discussing issues or topics relevant to them. It is important that you designate someone to take notes.

This is a simple visitation form that allows you to mix a number of partners together to gain some notoriety for your business retention and expansion program; it is a good training tool for new visitation representatives as well. It provides structure that allows you to gain valuable data and program recognition. It also allows you to cover varied businesses, including those outside of the program's normal focus, in a fixed amount of time. The data you receive is still important.

Whichever type of visitation is being performed, a thank you for doing business in the community is a must! All businesses could be doing business anywhere, but the one you are visiting is here. Community leaders should evaluate the business retention and expansion program over time and make continuous improvements as the economic and social environment changes.

Survey Says?

Everyone loves to take surveys, right? Not really. Surveys are a necessary part of the business retention and expansion program. As touched on in the discussion regarding visitation, one component of the program is to gather data that is relevant to healthy business operation in the community. To get any kind of traction with surveys, the subjects have to see the value in taking them; consideration of the time they will take is a factor.

It is also critical to define who the survey is aimed at. For business retention and expansion program surveys they must get to the right person. Typically, that person is a high-level manager, owner, or decision maker—someone who has to evaluate the business and most aspects of doing business on a daily basis. It should be someone with a vested interest in the success of the business who can articulate its ongoing needs. A common pitfall of surveys is that they end up on the desk of an assistant, front-line staff, or a company representative who does not really know the key issues or challenges the business is facing. This is true whether the survey is in the form of an email, postal delivered form, in-person, or by phone.

Response success is critical to provide valid and usable data, and numerous platforms are available. Surveyanyplace.com printed a list of survey methods and the estimated response rates. The blog compared in-person, mailed, emailed, online, telephone, and in-app surveys. It showed in-person with the highest rate of 57%, mailed surveys were at a close second of 50%, followed by a sharp decrease with emailed surveys dropping to around 30% (Lindemann, 2019). Again, it is important to note that surveys and the data provided are essential to providing quality solutions and feedback.

Surveys can be delivered electronically or by email, and this has become popular as a mass delivery tool. We get surveys in this fashion all the time. Even platforms like Facebook use this in-app where a friend can send a message and your responses to a series of questions will suggest what you would have been in the Wild West.

There are a number of challenges with electronic surveys. First, they can be easily ignored. With a simple press of the delete key, it is gone with no feedback. An important consideration in an electronic survey—as well as any survey—is its length. It may help to take the survey yourself or have the leadership team take it, time it out, and determine whether it is worth the time spent on it. The more concise it is, and the greater value the business perceives it to have, the more likely you are to get responses. What is the value of data received if 50 surveys are sent and you only receive one back? At least you will have learned that something was wrong in the way the survey was created or delivered, but little else.

A plus to email or electronic surveys

is that you can eliminate forms that are not completely filled out since it can be programmed to not tabulate unless the survey is completed to the end. This form of survey may also be self-tabulating, eliminating the need to perform additional data entry. Be aware it is still possible that the person who ends up completing the survey is not knowledgeable enough about the business to provide the information needed. So, follow-up is still important with this method of delivery.

The method of mailing a physical survey is still used to get to as many target businesses as possible. Depending on the source you look at, mailed surveys theoretically have a response rate second only to an in-person survey (Lindemann, 2019). Though mailed surveys may have fair results, the usual pitfalls still exist. A person not knowledgeable about key aspects of the business may be assigned to answer it. The survey may not be filled out completely and therefore may only have limited usefulness in data collection. Another problem of snail mail is that it may never reach its intended destination. Lastly, it will take staff time to enter the information collected.

Telephone surveys are another option. It will require staff time, both to conduct the phone calls and manually collect and enter the results. Timing is a distinct challenge. Unless the calls are made on a prearranged schedule there is no guarantee the right person will be available or have time when you place the call. This form of survey does allow you to verify you are interviewing the right person and offers the opportunity to ask follow-up questions that may be pertinent.

In the case of programs I have worked on, in-person surveying has netted the best results. A number of factors have made this a primary method of conducting surveys. First, you set appointments with the person you need to talk to around a scheduled time they designate, so you are likely to have their full attention and successfully get the information desired. The ability to read body language and inflection cues may allow you to identify issues that have greater significance to business. Meeting face-to-face allows you to have more complex discussions and provides the opportunity to ask follow-up questions on issues that may have greater relevance or need clarity. This is the best way to start or continue building a rapport with key businesspeople while ensuring a clear understanding of their concerns, needs, and commitment to the community.

Another option to surveying through a conversational means is to conduct roundtable meetings. Personal experience has led me to use this method often, due to limited time and resources and the chaotic challenges facing businesses in a time when they need to be able to express their needs and find critical resources in a quick time frame. Groups are brought together from same or similar industries to discuss pertinent relatable information. As a BRE tool it is effective in creating sector partnerships with the main point often focused on workforce issues.

However, if managed properly—working with the right champions and a promise of confidentiality by all participants—it can be used in creative and effective ways to still net quality data to answer questions and provide solutions. The COVID-19 crisis that emerged in March 2020 is an example of such an extraordinary time, when changes were so rapid, drastic, and unexpected that many business leaders needed someone to ask questions—not only to address immediate challenges but to know what questions to ask to meet the next unknown challenge of the time.

You can also host or participate in roundtable groups that have less of a business connection but a community connection. The conversational survey principle should still be followed, but the scope will likely be broader. An example is a recent forum discussion with active business owners in Arkansas's Polk County area, with a specific agenda of understanding the effects of COVID-19 on companies in a variety of industries. Some local elected officials participated as well. Once the ground rules were established the dialogue was very open and candid. It allowed us to get a snapshot of where they were through the progression of the pandemic. The nearly full participation provided data across a number of industries within the community. The information gained prompted the group to begin efforts to get out the message that they were open for business, just not as much as usual. This proved much more effective than an electronic survey promoted by multiple well-connected sources that netted only around a 10% return of surveys.

A note on surveys: They are as varied as practitioners. Design is always a topic that comes up when a group of BRE professionals or program leaders get together. It is critical that the information sought on the survey be relevant and have value to the business community it is intended to serve. It may be necessary to periodically review the survey information to make sure it provides useful information and is relevant to change that may occur within the community and business environment.

Managing the Data

Data collection is important to all business retention and expansion programs. It is the collation of the collected data that allows you to understand issues and draw conclusions on challenges for the area served by the program. Consistent data collected can be collated and disseminated to all parties to whom it is relevant. To that end, it will also be important to create or purchase a platform to enter and maintain the information collected. A few options are to create an information spreadsheet using software such as Excel, a database such as Access, or even customer relationship management software (CRM), of which there are a large number to choose from.

The managed data will allow stakeholders to look for solutions and make decisions on where to seek aid if necessary if resources are not readily available. The information collected from visits will be used to help determine follow-up solutions for those businesses that participated and may be used to assist businesses not yet contacted but sharing similar concerns.

Data collected from visits and meetings can also be used to identify trends in markets, labor pools, even be stratified to make determinations about locations within communities. By working with other developer groups, community leaders, and civic organizations, the BRE program can use generalized data to assist in other aspects of the community such as transportation challenges, internet dead zones, growth areas, housing issues, or any number of factors that make a community successful.

Because of the nature of the information being collected it is important that you follow the confidentiality terms you committed to. Be cognizant of information that could easily identify the business that shared it. Helping businesses in your community keep a competitive edge is a primary goal of this program. Integrity is essential to encourage business to participate and to keep open opportunities for future follow-up.

Follow-up to Strengthen the Community

Follow-up in a business retention and expansion program anywhere follows similar protocols. After a visitation and input of the resulting data, it goes to a review. The review of the information collected from business visits is used to establish that all questions got answered and to determine what if any critical follow-up is necessary for the health of the business. Reviews are performed by an action team or task force. Action teams should include representatives of organizations and individuals that provide services and tools to assist businesses with identified action items (Jacobs, 2016, p. 1). A task force approach can also be used with a group made up of business leaders, development professionals, local officials, educators, and key community leaders who are then divided into smaller teams to review and address issues (Tweeten & Barefield, 2017, pp. 15–20).

Typically, information reviewed is categorized using a flag system utilizing the colors green, yellow, and red. Green indicates the business is healthy with few or no issues or problems identified during the visit. Yellow means that some potential concerns were discussed or uncovered and some response is necessary, though nothing suggests the business might move or its operations are hampered in the community. A red flag, however, identifies an issue critical to the business visited. There are a number of ways to determine how to respond to visitations, but that will be a product of your program design. Whether reports will be presented to an action team or shared through another process, it is particularly important to address and respond to those items identified as yellow or red.

Though all identified questions and concerns should be addressed, a red flag item requires a quick response representing an issue that is or will shortly lead to a crisis for that business. Remembering the importance of preserving confidentiality, the red flag issue is presented to the appropriate action team or task force. Once the team works through the concern and discerns possible solutions related to the issue the solutions should be presented to the designated program leader. An assessment of resources necessary to address the issue needs to be completed, after which the program leader or other appropriate designee can provide options to the business.

Communication is key—between program members, resource providers, and the business. Clear and concise options may make the difference in a business's future. One possible by-product of review and follow-up is creation of a resource guide. By looking at local issues and concerns and then working with a variety of agencies and organizations—private, public, and nonprofit—your program should develop a catalog of resources and services available to your community. The most important takeaway to follow-up is just that: Be sure someone responds to each business visited, whether responding to a flagged issue or just sending a thank-you for their time. It will go a long way to promoting your program and showing value to those who take the time to engage.

Steps to Getting Started

We have covered a lot of ground regarding business retention and expansion, and now you have to make some decisions. Do you move forward with your own program? If so, how and with whom? To what end?

The steps below are actions I recommend and have used launching BRE projects of varied scope and size. The most obvious first step is to act. Whether it is meeting with the economic development circle or local leadership team, you have to start the discussion. Creating a business retention and expansion program will take time and some level of resources. The resources available will likely be a factor in determining the initial depth and scope of the program. Businesses today operate in a competitive world economy. Waiting for someone else will not get it done. Local businesses need you to care about their business and to provide opportunity for them to stay and grow with your community.

My first recommendation to you is

recruit a BRE professional—or at least someone with experience in these types of programs. Next, identify key stakeholders and champions who are committed to the well-being and future of the community. They should be respected in the community, have a sizable network of friends and peers, and be willing to promote the program. Select people who are willing to participate, put their time and energy into the project, and use discretion when necessary to push a positive public agenda to help create excitement around the program. It is my recommendation that this group be limited in size—small enough to make agile decisions and large enough to diversely represent a majority of the community. Having lead team members with different circles of influence should help with outreach efforts to communicate the value of the program and identify a wide range of resources that could benefit the business community.

Once the champions or leadership team is established the work begins: determine a vision and mission of the program. I suggest that the groups I work with identify three focus points that should have value to local businesses and work around these. Branding is important since this will make the program more recognizable and easier to promote with a common theme. Uniformity of information about the program will be important when it is new and light a fire when things start to stall. (It happens.) You will probably find that formulating the vision, mission, and branding will take a few meetings to get the brainstorming juices flowing, and that is OK. This will most likely be a new concept to the group and will take time for them to grasp. I have found that even people that work with businesses or in development for a living struggle to pinpoint where to begin.

Begin promoting the program: first in circles of influence and then to more groups throughout the community, particularly the business community. I am currently working with a city where that group decided to start by holding a question-and-answer session with key business leaders to get input and make sure the direction of the project had common value. You could hold a town hall type meeting or speak with chamber and business organizations in the community to get a buzz started. However you begin, expect feedback and work with it.

Determine the structure of your program. The group will need to develop training materials for new team members as they come on board. Training should be provided for each aspect of the program with particular attention and practice given to the visitation team. This should include how to complete a survey conversationally. Not many people like to answer questions while the interviewer checks boxes. I also remind our teams to ask permission to call or email back if they have other questions. Surprisingly, that gets positive results.

Consider how you will divide the work and what each team will be responsible for. Keep in mind, the leadership team sets the scope for each team. As part of this process, determine how information will be communicated—from leadership to visitation to data entry to follow-up and so on. The structure of the program will vary based on available resources. Decide on the number of members per team and how many of each type of team you might have. This will affect the number of businesses you can reach in a given period of time and how often to do visitations. Be realistic as you set these goals.

Agree on what you should get out of every visit and on a consistent, reliable way to retain and track the information. Set confidentiality parameters and clearly communicate this to businesses. You may want to create a confidentiality document that both parties sign. Create a survey that fits your community and that will represent a good value to the businesses that participate while respecting their time. Survey questions have to be meaningful and some—such as pay, turnover, shortages, and the like—will be uncomfortable. Some of these questions, however, need to be asked to ascertain the health of the business and identify what they need assistance with.

Establish protocols for follow-up and flag issues. Decide who will reach out to resource partners and who will report back to the company in concern. Set how the program staff will share information to other entities in the community and how the message will be presented to the general public. After all, the health of local business should be of interest to all the citizens of the community.

Be sure to tell your story. Share successes, small wins, and community-change events. People are more likely to participate if they feel the program is making a difference; if they are not part of the program team it may not be evident that progress is being made. Take pictures and post them on relevant social media platforms as well as community websites. Issue press releases and hold open meetings to allow the public to understand the project and how it affects the whole community. Publicity may invite encouragement and insights from local businesses and leaders. This can be helpful and give you connections to resources when things bog down.

A concept shared by a number of developers is that a community is either growing or dying. There is no neutral for a community because opportunity will go where it is wanted and can prosper. Make sure businesses in the community know they are important and appreciated. Ensure the sustainability of your BRE program by having full community support. If local business and citizens know there is a program that supports continued growth, they will share the news, which will help to promote the story that yours is a healthy business community.

Case Study
Grants Pass, Oregon

In 1996, the city of Grants Pass, Oregon, did not have an economic development plan. A newly hired economic development coordinator, along with the city manager, was assigned the task of writing one and decided that the core of the new plan would be business retention and expansion. At the same time, the local chamber of commerce reconvened a standing committee that had been dormant for many years—a committee that happened to be called the Business Retention and Expansion (BR&E) Committee. The city's economic development coordinator was appointed chair of the newly organized BR&E Committee.

Through his research, he came across the BR&E program out of the University of Minnesota. After looking at a variety of options, the committee decided to pursue the University of Minnesota Extension BR&E visitation model. After training by the University of Minnesota Extension, he was certified by BREI (Business Retention and Expansion International) to manage a BR&E program. He then facilitated the program locally as a joint effort by the city and the local chamber of commerce.

With a population of just under 80,000, the BR&E program conducted 100 interviews in the first two years. The businesses represented a cross-section of both the Grants Pass Urban Area (about 75%) and the rest of the county (about 25%), as well as a cross-section of business sectors within each.

The Project

The City of Grants Pass and the local chamber of commerce have conducted and completed business visitations every three years since 1999. In 1999, the first round of surveys quantified pent-up demand in the community for additional industrial real estate. Several local businesses needed to expand immediately. The committee used their knowledge of land available in the area and served as a conduit between the businesses and the landowners to facilitate the development of an industrial park. Because it was a private development, the developers had been hesitant to build without guaranteed buyers. The BR&E committee went to the developers with the confirmation that five local businesses needed the land fast. The committee served as an important link between the businesses and the developers—a link that had not existed prior to the project.

Results

Even though three businesses purchased land initially, the interest of one major business triggered the rest of the development. A local electronics manufacturer became the first tenant of the industrial park less than two years after the BR&E

visits were completed. This manufacturer, which had operated in the community for more than 20 years, described its expansion needs during the BR&E visits and expressed a need for help in getting the expansion done. The park made their business expansion goals possible. Since their expansion, they not only have a new facility and dramatically increased efficiency but they have doubled their employment to more than 200 workers.

The company's decision to locate in the industrial park allowed the committee to leverage grants to get the necessary infrastructure built. Other businesses began to follow when the economy picked up in 2002 and 2003. In the first two phases 18 lots have been sold in the industrial park. All of the businesses employ fewer than 200 employees, and now there is a mixture of businesses in the park both new to Grants Pass and previously existing in the community.

The industrial park was perhaps Josephine County BR&E program's most visible success, and it helped the program secure two awards. In 1999, the program won the Governor's Sustainable Oregon Award, which recognizes community-level, grassroots programs that sustain Oregon's quality of life. Then in 2001, the Grants Pass/Josephine County program won the Business Retention and Expansion International (BREI) award for Outstanding Community BR&E Program.

For more information about the project see https://extension.umn.edu/retaining-community-businesses/retaining-businesses-case-studies-and-stories

Resources to Jump Start a Program

Business Retention Expansion International (BREI) is an organization with the primary focus of cultivating BRE programs. The organization provides training and certifications in business retention and expansion. BREI has a membership across the globe, but the majority of members practice in the United States and Canada. More information can be found at their website: https://brei.org/

International Economic Development Council (IEDC) is a nonprofit, nonpartisan membership organization serving economic developers. The mission stated on their website is to "provide leadership and excellence in economic development for our communities, members, and partners." IEDC offers courses in business retention and expansion. More information about the IEDC is available at https://www.iedconline.org/

A number of extension service offices also offer BRE support and technical assistance. North Dakota State University Extension Service, Mississippi State University Extension Service, University of Minnesota Extension, and University of Florida IFAS Extension are a few that have contributed to the promotion of BRE programs.

Information on the Business Walk mentioned earlier in the chapter can be found at http://www.businessfirstdaytonregion.com/node/249. This is a Business-First! example from the Dayton, Ohio area; the city of Quesnel, British Columbia has an example at https://www.quesnel.ca/sites/default/files/uploads/reports/business_walks_2016.pdf

References

Deane, M.T. (2020, February 28). Top 6 reasons new businesses fail. *Investopedia.* https://www.investopedia.com/financial-edge/1010/top-6-reasons-new-businesses-fail.aspx

Farnsworth, D., Clark, J.L. & Cothran, H. (n.d.). *Business retention and expansion (BRE) programs: Characteristics of successful BRE programs.* University of Florida IFAS Extension.

Jacobs, P.A. (2016). *Business retention & expansion program manual.* Halifax Partnership. https://businessretention.files.wordpress.com/2017/12/bre-program-manual-ver-1-3-nov-2016.pdf

Lindemann, N. (2019, August 8). *What's the average survey response rate?* SurveyAnyplace. https://surveyanyplace.com/average-survey-response-rate/

Small business profile. (2019). Office of Advocacy, U.S. Small Business Association.

Teamwork Arkansas. (2005.). *Business retention and expansion guide.* Entergy Arkansas Office of Economic Development. https://bowenisland.civicweb.net/document/59000/Business_Retention_Expansion_Guidebook.pdf?handle=946CFBCAAF474008A24CF2ABAFE7331A

Tweeten, K. & Barefield, A. (2017, September). *Business retention and expansion visitation fundamentals.* North Dakota State University Extension Service Center for Community Vitality. https://www.ag.ndsu.edu/publications/community-development/business-retention-and-expansion-visitation-fundamentals-1

What is BR&E? (2018). Business Retention & Expansion International. https://brei.org/what-is-bre/

Community and Economic Development Finance

Toby Rittner, DFCP

Creating a remarkable community with sustainable infrastructure and the ability to influence its growth takes fiscal management and insightful risk assessment strategies. Learn to maintain full-cost funding and budgeting for long-term success.

Learning Outcomes

- Participants will understand the role of finance within the community and economic development process.

- Participants will explore community and economic development funding tools.

- Participants will learn how to establish a local funding team.

Development finance is the effort of local communities to support, encourage, and catalyze economic growth. It is a tool to help make a project or deal successful and in turn create a benefit for the long-term health of a community. This benefit is the economic growth that can take place through public and private investment in infrastructure, business, and industry.

Development finance offers a potential solution to the challenges of the local economic, business, and industrial environment. To use development finance tools effectively, practitioners must possess an understanding of the myriad programs, resources, and terminology that exist in this field.

Economic development professionals play an important role as the bridge between government and business. They direct the use of precious public resources, inform policy decisions about how resources are allocated, and act as catalysts for important projects.

What Does Development Finance Include?

Development finance tools come in a variety of forms. These tools include loans, equity, tax abatements, and tax credits. They also include the offer of a guarantee, collateral, or some other form of credit enhancement within the context of a complex financing package. Development finance may include gap financing, which often makes the difference between a project that is contemplated and one that reaches fruition. Development finance tools may also include the remediation of environmental concerns as well as incentives, grants, or other resources for businesses and entrepreneurs.

Development finance is a proactive approach toward finance intended to assist economic development projects. It leverages valuable public resources to support significant private sector investment. Development finance also involves capturing capacity and advantages throughout the community and beyond geographic boundaries. It is dedicated to building partnerships and establishing collaborative approaches to solve complex development challenges. In doing so, development finance helps to solve the needs of business, industry, developers, and investors, while also contributing to a community's long-term health and goals.

What Does Development Finance Not Include?

Development finance comes with accountability measures; it is not a "free ride" for businesses in need of assistance. The use of public resources should be tied to performance measurements and project achievements. Development finance programs should not compete with programs offered by private financial institutions, because this could create conflict, an uneven playing field, and a lack of cooperation among stakeholders. Rather, public financing should complement and enhance the offerings of the private sector.

Public contributions towards development finance should bring commensurate public rewards. Unabashed subsidies that provide public contribution while requiring too little private commitment are not considered good practice by professionals.

Balancing public risk against public reward is perhaps the most difficult component of this process. Development professionals, however, have established methodologies to determine the appropriate amount of public financing that should be contributed to a project or a business. Such methodologies help the public achieve a maximum return on its investment.

Development finance requires a rational, thoughtful, and strategic response to economic needs and challenges. Many communities struggle with sudden economic adjustments due to plant closings, corporate relocations, or business expansions. Community leaders are placed under considerable pressure to address these challenges quickly. To present a thoughtful response to such challenges, development finance must include long-term strategic thinking.

Why is Development Finance Important?

Development finance is critical to economic development because it has the potential to make or break a project. Businesses need access to financial resources to complete a project or deal. Whether the funds are used for site acquisition or startup capital, nearly all projects hinge on the borrower's ability to leverage convenient sources of financing. Development finance may offer a less expensive type of financing than conventional private financing.

Development finance can help businesses generate working capital and invest in their growth. It can help developers achieve an acceptable return on investment (ROI) in a given project. It can help communities develop infrastructure, jobs, and amenities. In pursuing a development finance strategy, it is essential to balance the needs of industry with the needs of the community.

A proposal to use development finance tools may act as a catalyst for development led by the private sector, regardless of whether or not public financing is actually utilized. For instance, the creation of a tax increment financing (TIF) district can prompt an increase in investment based on the speculation that real estate values will increase in the area—even if the municipality never issues a bond or finances a deal. Such increased investment may cause real estate values to rise, thus bringing in additional tax revenues in areas targeted for redevelopment. Furthermore, the increase in investment spurred by the use or perceived use of development finance tools may ultimately help foster community buy-in.

Principles of Development Finance

There are five key principles of development finance.

1. Finance, generally speaking, is agnostic to your project. Projects are important, but finance cares mostly about one key question: How are you going to repay your debt?

2. Finance wants to know all the details. While agnostic to the project, finance wants to know how you will use the money lent to you. Can you define your project? For example:

- What is the actual project?
- What is the timeline?
- How much will the project cost?
- Who are the customers or target market?
- Do you have land control?
- What are the alternatives?
- What are the expectations?

3. Finance is about identifying sources of revenue. Remember, finance wants to know: How are you going to repay your debt? So it is important to find revenue streams, such as rents, fees, appropriations, equity, donations, grants, sales, or assessments.

4. Financing a project requires that you embrace the alternatives. Development finance is very difficult, and the project you envision simply may not be supported by the sources and uses available. Embrace the alternatives early in the process. You may find that you can meet your goals by being open to new realities and new partners.

5. Development finance is all about identifying barriers to capital, removing those barriers, and then identifying all the sources of capital that can contribute to the project financing. So, know your sources. Sources of funding and finance include:

- municipal bonds
- industrial development bonds
- 501(c)3 bonds
- exempt facilities bonds
- tax increment finance
- New Markets Tax Credits
- revolving loan funds
- EB-5 Immigrant Investor Program
- Opportunity Zones
- property assessed clean energy
- special assessment
- Linked Deposit programs
- mezzanine funds

- grants
- tax abatements
- seed and venture capital
- historic tax credits
- many more…

Trends in Development Finance

The development finance industry ebbs and flows with the economy and is often subject to the same market forces as traditional lending tools. Development finance agencies take on a variety of roles, including:

- issuing bonds directly or acting as a conduit issuer;
- providing direct loans;
- providing loan guarantees or other collateral support;
- providing grants;
- providing technical assistance;
- serving as developer or development partner.

Despite all of this, according to research from the Council of Development Finance Agencies (CDFA), 50% of all finance agencies allocate less than 20% of their actual budget to financing development (Rittner, 2009). This is due to a variety of reasons, including the complexity of programs, a general lack of resources for administering them, and insufficient staff education. In the most extreme cases, certain tools may lack political support.

Development finance is a complex undertaking. These tools require a considerable amount of knowledge and training, and in many communities the resources to educate all of the parties involved do not exist. Lack of education and training is a major hindrance to the development finance process, and it can create project obstacles and legal problems in the long run.

Education is the most critical strategy to make these tools easier to use and understand. Successful agencies build their programs by educating staff and leadership. Because education requires an investment of resources, development finance agencies must be mindful of allocating funds for this purpose.

The Financing Spectrum

Every economic development transaction presents different challenges. For instance, large-scale industrial development requires a different financing approach when compared to small business development. Typically, development finance is broken down into a spectrum of approaches. An understanding of this spectrum will allow development finance agencies to address the needs of established industries, large real estate development projects, small businesses, and individual entrepreneurs.

Some financing options, such as a revolving loan fund, may address a variety of needs and clients. To be effective, however, most development finance efforts must be tailored to a specific need or project. For instance, real estate development does not require the use of startup capital such as seed or venture capital funding. On the other hand, an early-stage entrepreneur is not likely to benefit from bond financing.

This guide will explore the spectrum of development finance tools. Understanding this spectrum is critical to maximizing the development finance resources available in a community.

Building the Development Finance Toolbox

Hundreds of development finance programs exist at the federal, state, and local levels. These programs have been created over the past two centuries to address the financing needs of business, industry, real estate, housing, and environmental and community development entities.

Individually, none of these programs is a silver-bullet solution to the economic development challenges such entities face. The toolbox approach to development finance brings together the best of these financing concepts and techniques to provide a comprehensive response to capital and resource needs. The toolbox approach offers programs and resources that harness the full spectrum of financing options. This approach requires a commitment to public–private partnerships and the creation of niche programs to assist different types of industries and enterprises. Whether assisting large-scale industrial development projects or small, microenterprise business development, the toolbox approach is designed to help numerous types of users and maximize opportunities for growth in the local economy.

Economic development professionals have one of the most difficult job descriptions in local government: to catalyze investment, promote opportunity for new and expanding businesses, and create jobs. The toolbox approach recognizes the financing challenges that economic development projects face and seeks to provide realistic and comprehensive solutions.

A broad array of financing programs currently exists across the country, yet in most cases they are underutilized. The use of tax credit programs is an example. According to CDFA research, less than 5% of finance agencies frequently employ the use of state and federal tax credit programs (Rittner, 2009). Yet these programs represent the most abundant financing source in the country, offering targeted and tailored programs to address financing needs.

Using the toolbox approach allows economic development professionals to take a comprehensive approach to financing. The toolbox pulls together a variety of programs and offers different tools for a range of users and projects. The toolbox also collects funding sources at the federal, state, and local-government levels—and within the private sector—in one place. This comprehensive approach toward the use of public resources is more likely to attract business, investment, and growth to a community.

Understanding the development finance spectrum is critical to maximizing the resources available in a community. The toolbox approach addresses this spectrum by breaking down dozens of financing options into several core areas.

Bedrock Tools: Bond Finance

Bonds are the bedrock of public development finance. Bond finance dates back to the 19th century, with the deferral tax exemption included in the country's first federal tax code. In its simplest form, a bond is a debt or a loan incurred by a governmental entity. Bonds are issued and sold to the investing public, and the proceeds are typically made available to finance the costs of a capital project. If the bonds are being issued for the benefit of a nongovernmental borrower, the proceeds are often loaned to such a borrower, and the borrower then makes loan payments corresponding to when principal and interest are due on the bonds. Bondholders receive interest over the term of the bonds, and such interest is often exempt from federal, state, and local income taxes. The tax-exempt status of certain bonds makes them an attractive investment option for investors.

There are two types of tax-exempt bonds: government bonds (GOs) and qualified private activity bonds (PABs). Government bonds are intended to address the traditional infrastructure needs of the nation. GOs may be used for many public purposes (e.g., highways, schools, bridges, sewers, jails, parks, and government equipment and buildings), and their debt service requirements are met by levying taxes on the general public. Facilities financed by GOs are not permitted to be significantly used, operated, controlled, or owned by private entities. Conversely, PABs permit a larger degree of private sector involvement and are used to address numerous development finance needs identified by Congress and state and local governments. PABs drive projects involving both the public and private sectors by passing along the low-cost interest benefit—generated by the tax-exempt status of PABs—to private borrowers. While the language governing the usage of GOs is fairly straightforward, the language governing PAB regulations and uses is far more complicated. The Internal Revenue Code (IRC) permits the financing of several types of projects using qualified PABs, although they may be used partially or entirely for private purposes.

Qualified PABs generally include:

- industrial development bonds
- 501(c)(3) bonds
- exempt facility bonds
- qualified redevelopment bonds
- Aggie Bonds
- green bonds

Industrial Development Bonds

Small Issue Industrial Development Bonds (IDBs) are also referred to as Small Issue Manufacturing Bonds or Industrial Development Bonds. These bonds are the single most actively used bond tool for financing the manufacturing sector and are a key economic development tool for many states. IDBs are issued for qualified manufacturing projects, with a total bond issuance limit of $10 million. These bonds can support expansion and investment in existing manufacturing facilities, as well as the development of new facilities and the purchase of new machinery and equipment.

501(c)(3) Bonds

501(c)(3) bonds finance projects owned and used by not-for-profit corporations that qualify for exemption under Section 501(c)(3) of the IRC. Due to the relative affordability of this type of financing, 501(c)(3) bonds have gained popularity over the past several years. Organizations using 501(c)(3) bonds may include universities and private colleges, continuing care facilities, independent and charter schools, cultural organizations, hospitals, religious or charitable groups, and scientific organizations.

Exempt Facility Bonds

Exempt facility bonds finance a wide variety of projects, including airports, docks, mass-commuting facilities (such as high-speed rail), water and sewage facilities, solid waste disposal facilities, qualified low-income residential rental projects, facilities that furnish electric energy or gas, qualified public educational facilities, and qualified highway or surface-freight transfer facilities. Exempt facility bonds have a wide scope of use, and implementation varies by state or local government.

Qualified Redevelopment Bonds

Infrastructure projects that do not qualify for government bonds may qualify for tax-exempt financing if they meet several tests. For instance, in many cases, the proceeds must fund redevelopment in designated areas of blight. These bonds are typically issued for projects that involve special district financing, such as tax increment financing (TIF).

Aggie Bonds

Aggie Bonds are small issue bonds and exist in many states to support agricultural investment. Aggie Bonds provide an attractive, affordable source of capital for first-time farmers looking to invest in a new business venture. These programs are often managed by the state agriculture department or similar authority.

Green Bonds

Businesses and governments issue green bonds to raise funds for a range of environmental projects. The issuer has to ensure that the proceeds from the sale of the bonds are invested in green projects such as renewable energy, energy efficiency, and projects leading to reduced carbon emissions.

Bond Players

The bond finance process is complex and requires considerable oversight. In each transaction, varieties of players serve critical roles to ensure that the process is effective, efficient, and conducted within the scope of the law. Almost all bonds issued by state and local political subdivisions are accompanied by the approving legal opinion of a recognized bond counsel law firm. Some of the key bond players are:

- **Bond issuer:** an organization that registers, distributes, and sells a bond on the primary bond market. A bond issuer can be a private organization or a government.

- **Bond counsel:** an attorney or law firm retained by the issuer to give a legal opinion. The bond counsel's approving legal opinion gives investors assurance as to the validity, security, and tax-exempt status of the bond.

- **Underwriter:** an investment bank or group that agrees to purchase an entire security issue for a specific price, usually for resale to others

- **Trustee:** a bank designated by an issuer of bonds to act as the custodian of funds and official representative of the bondholders

- **Municipal advisor:** a consultant who advises the issuer on matters pertinent to the issue, such as structure, timing, marketing, fairness of pricing, terms, and bond ratings

- **Rating organization:** an entity that provides a rating that gives indications of credit quality

Bond Ratings

Bond ratings are determined by nationally recognized rating agencies such as Standard & Poor's, Moody's, and Fitch to indicate an issuer's credit strength in a particular financing. The rating in effect speaks to the probability that bond investors will be paid in full and on time by the borrower. Bond ratings play a very important role in the issuance process because they determine the levels and interest rates at which bonds may be issued. Although each of the three major credit rating services may weigh each of the following general categories of credit analysis somewhat differently, they all rely on these basic criteria:

- debt factors
- economic factors
- administrative/governmental factors
- fiscal/financial performance factors

These fundamental factors apply to all types of bonds, including both government and PABs. Although bonds do not legally require a rating, market circumstances compel most issuers to have their large debt issues rated. Investors use the bond ratings to analyze the degree of risk associated with purchasing various public securities.

How Bonds Are Sold

New issues of municipal bonds are sold by one of three methods: (1) competitive; (2) negotiated; or (3) private placement. After bonds are sold, most municipal bonds are traded in the secondary market. Unlike the corporate and stock markets, the municipal bond secondary market(s) are not formal. There is no institution such as the New York State Exchange where sale offerings are publicly listed. Rather, the municipal secondary market rests on hundreds of broker dealers nationwide who serve as agents for the buying and selling of previously sold bonds, an over-the-counter market.

In relation to economic development efforts, the bonds outlined above represent the most concrete, readily available source of public finance. When issuing bonds, coordination among and between the appropriate bond players throughout the process is critical to a project's success. Moreover, PAB use has increased exponentially during the past two decades, and today they serve as the primary source for financing many types of projects, including infrastructure, industrial development, and urban development.

Targeted Tools: Tax Increment Finance, Special Assessment Districts

Targeted tools are the second most common form of development finance in the United States. This area of finance focuses on geographical tax treatments that drive development, redevelopment, and neighborhood improvement. The primary tools in this part of the toolbox are special assessment and tax increment finance. This section will predominantly speak to tax increment finance.

Tax increment financing (TIF) is referred to in a variety of ways throughout the country. These terms include tax allocation district (TAD–Georgia), tax increment reinvestment zone (TIRZ–Texas), community reinvestment area (CRA–Florida) and economic redevelopment and growth grant (ERGG–New Jersey). Generally, however, TIFs adhere to a similar structure and function in a similar fashion, regardless of geography. Today, 48 states and the District of Columbia employ TIF tools, with rules and regulations varying by state.

A TIF district is a mechanism for capturing the future tax benefits of real estate improvements in order to pay for their present cost. It can be used to channel funding toward improvements in distressed or underdeveloped areas where development would not otherwise occur.

Tax increment finance is a popular development finance tool generally used to address blight, promote neighborhood stability, and inspire district-oriented development. While each state's TIF statute is different, common policy goals and objectives exist. These intentions include blight elimination, something discussed in nearly every state's statute, and infrastructure additions and improvements.

A TIF district is often used to advance economic development priorities, including:

- guiding public finance dollars toward targeted investment and development;
- developing industry niches and opening new markets for services that do not exist in a given geographic area;

- supporting overall development within a specific geographic area;
- reusing existing infrastructure and cleaning up polluted or brownfield land; and
- creating or retaining jobs and supporting industrial development.

A TIF district is a powerful tool that can address many needs in a community. It is often used to encourage development, eliminate blight, address environmental issues, and facilitate adaptive reuse. TIF uses the increased property and/or sales taxes generated by a new development to finance costs related to that particular development. These costs may include public infrastructure, land acquisition, relocation, demolition, utilities, debt service, and planning costs. A TIF district may also be used for a variety of other improvements, including:

- sewer expansion and repair
- park improvements
- bridge construction and repair
- street lighting
- property and building acquisition
- environmental remediation
- street construction and expansion

Due Diligence & Transparency

The due diligence process is one of the most important elements in the use of TIF and should be considered throughout the decision making and financing process. Some local governments fail to conduct a thorough financial and legal analysis and find difficulties in project completion as a result of these actions. With a solid process for vetting and evaluating TIF projects, however, the local government can minimize conflict and increase community participation in project fulfilment. Local governments should implement a transparent and thorough due diligence process. This includes closely examining the financial risk the local government will bear as well as the legal requirements of the state enabling legislation. Depending on the state statute and the structure of specific TIF financings, local governments may face a variety of risk factors, including:

- potential for tax revenues to fall short of projections;
- project delays or failure to complete projects;
- restrictions on investment of bond proceeds;
- limitations on tax-exempt financings;

- restrictions on the cost categories for which TIF funds can be used;
- ability of other taxing jurisdictions to claim a portion of TIF revenues to reimburse their costs;
- costs incurred without offsetting tax revenues; and
- negative political fallout and consequences.

Engaging quality bond counsel and financial experts throughout the process can mitigate these risks. In addition, fully understanding the TIF laws before applying the tool will help keep legal issues from developing further into the process. While TIF can finance a variety of improvements, it does have limitations that should be understood.

The "But For" Analysis

Some states require that a "But For" test be met before a TIF deal can be approved. Such a test shows that "but for" the proposed level of TIF assistance and given timetable for the project, development at the proposed scale would not occur. This type of analysis is a strongly recommended best practice for TIF programs in all states for the following reasons:

- keeps the purpose of the public investment clear
- promotes judicious use of public dollars
- maintains strong accountability to the affected taxing jurisdictions
- puts limitations on tax-exempt financing usage

Community Education and Engagement Process

In most states, the TIF process requires local governments to hold open and public discussions. In order for a local government to use TIF to its fullest potential, it is essential to educate the community. TIF is a powerful tool and the process must be conducted in an open and thoughtful fashion. There are a number of areas that the local governments should consider as part of the education and engagement process, including building consensus, identifying stakeholders, media, and communication and marketing.

Accountability

The responsibility of implementation of TIF ultimately rests with the powers of local government. This power yields an accountability factor that cannot be ignored or set aside for the sake of priorities, headlines, or an eagerness to complete the projects. Local governments that follow the recommended practices for due diligence and transparency will find it easier to comply with accountability requirements.

In each of these categories of qualified PABs, bonds must meet the specific requirements of the IRC. These tests can be complex, and they require a clear understanding before bonds may be issued in order to ensure tax-exempt status. In relation to economic development efforts, the bonds outlined above represent the most concrete, readily available source of public finance.

Investment Tools: Tax Credits, Opportunity Zones, and EB-5

Tax Credits

Tax credit programs allow businesses and investors to claim tax credits for committing resources to a project or business. Several different types of tax credit programs exist at the federal and state levels to encourage investments in redevelopment projects, affordable housing, specific industries, and communities of all sizes.

Tax credits directly reduce a taxpayer's tax liability, making them a very desirable and effective tool. They can be used in urban, rural, and suburban communities, and in some cases on a regional basis. They can also provide a targeted impact by addressing many different community sectors, such as low-income neighborhoods, historic districts, and underserved markets that present opportunities for new investment.

There are three primary federal tax credit programs: New Markets Tax Credits, Historic Rehabilitation Tax Credits, and Low-Income Housing Tax Credits. There are also numerous state tax credit programs available.

In order to receive a tax credit, an investor must first demonstrate that an investment has been made. Such a resource commitment could be an investment in a brick- and-mortar real estate project or a cash investment in a business. The distributor of the tax credit is authorized to issue credit based on the actual outlay of resources as evidenced by the investor. Tax credits can be used for several purposes in development projects: to provide an increased internal rate of return for investors, to reduce the interest rates on a particular financing package, and perhaps most importantly, to provide a repayment method for investors in place of cash. In the latter case, the credits can often be sold on the secondary market to generate income.

Opportunity Zones

Opportunity Zones, created as a result of the passage of the Tax Cuts and Jobs Act, are low-income census tracts eligible to use tax incentives to encourage long-term investments in Zone assets and property. Approximately 8,700+ census tracts have been designated as Opportunity Zones in all states, the District of Columbia, and U.S. territories (Community Development Financial Institutions Fund, n.d.).

To receive investment in local businesses or real estate projects, an Opportunity Zone must attract equity investments from Opportunity Funds, which are capitalized by investors who have realized gains on a recent transaction. Those investors can defer their federal capital gains taxes from that transaction for up to 10 years as long as 90% of the assets in an Opportunity Fund are directly invested in qualified projects in Opportunity Zones. Further, if the Opportunity Fund experiences any gains during that 10-year period, those gains are fully exempted from federal capital gains tax.

Opportunity Zones offer communities exciting new ways to access capital, especially into areas that have received disinvestment for many years or decades. Understanding how to use capital from Opportunity Funds is critical to realizing a successful investment strategy that drives both economic and social impact directly into communities and neighborhoods. Because Opportunity Funds can be used to support both business and real estate projects in Opportunity Zones, it is important for communities to be proactive in identifying potential investments and coordinating with multiple stakeholders.

EB-5

The EB-5 program is a federally authorized visa category created by Congress in 1990. The primary concept is to encourage foreign investment in job-creating U.S. economic development projects or companies in return for a U.S. green card. These projects or companies must create or retain 10 full-time jobs in the States, and a minimum investment of $1 million is required. This investment can be reduced to $500,000 if it is made in a high unemployment or rural area. Once the investment in a qualifying project or company has been made, the investor receives a conditional green card for two years. After two years, the investor must prove that their investment has been maintained and that the 10 jobs continue to exist. At this point, the conditional status is removed.

EB-5 projects are typically financed through regional centers, which can accept the investment from the green card-seeking investor. The U.S. government sets aside 10,000 green cards each year for foreign investors participating through designated regional centers. The centers invest in projects that meet all of the program criteria. Using the EB-5 program is not simple, and there are significant investment and timing rules that must be followed. These rules can mean the difference between an investor receiving a green card or being deported. It is vital that participants consult and work only with reputable and qualified regional centers, immigration lawyers, and project finance experts. EB-5 financing is available in every state and city in the country.

Access to Capital Lending Tools: Revolving Loan Funds

A revolving loan fund (RLF) is a gap financing measure primarily used for development and expansion of small businesses. It is a self-replenishing pool of money, utilizing interest and principal payments on old loans to issue new ones. While the majority of RLFs support local businesses, some target specific areas such as healthcare, minority business development, and environmental cleanup.

A revolving loan fund provides access to a flexible source of capital that can be used in combination with more conventional sources. Often, the RLF is a bridge between the amount the borrower can obtain on the private market and the amount needed to start or sustain a business. For example, a borrower may obtain 60 to 80% of project financing from other sources.

Quality RLFs issue loans at market or otherwise competitive and attractive rates. Many RLF studies have shown that access to capital and flexibility in collateral and terms is more important to borrowers than lower-than-market interest rates. RLF programs should be built on sound interest-rate practices and not perceived as free or easy sources of financing. RLFs must be able to generate enough of an interest rate return to replenish the fund for future loan allocations. With competitive rates and flexible terms, a RLF provides access to new financing sources for the borrower while lowering overall risk for participating institutional lenders. Typical uses for RLF loans include:

- operating capital
- acquisition of land and buildings
- new construction
- facade and building renovation
- landscape and property improvements
- machinery and equipment

Loan Characteristics

Loan terms vary according to the use of funds. A loan used for working capital, for instance, may range from 3 to 5 years, while loans for equipment are up to 10 years and real estate loans may last 15 to 20 years. It is important that terms are fixed to the useful life of the asset financed.

Loan amounts range from small ($1,000 to $10,000) to mid-sized ($25,000 to $75,000), with larger ($100,000 to $250,000 and up) amounts available when the borrower has secured a substantial sum from private lenders.

Capitalizing a Loan Fund

Initial funding, or capitalization, of a revolving loan fund usually comes from a combination of public sources, such as local, state, and federal governments, and private ones such as financial institutions and philanthropic organizations. Funding acquired for capitalization is usually the equivalent of a grant; it does not need to be paid back. Most revolving loan funds have at least one local public source for capitalization combined with other sources. If capitalization is exclusively local, the RLF may have greater flexibility in lending, as state and federal involvement tends to impose restrictions that may not fit local business needs.

State and local governments often use one or a combination of the following to capitalize an RLF: tax setasides, general obligation bonds, direct appropriations from the state legislature, annual dues from participating counties or municipalities, and funds directed from the state lottery.

The federal government is another common source of capitalization. Communities may apply for funding from the United States Department of Agriculture (via the Rural Economic and Community Development Administration), Housing and Urban Development (via Community Development Block Grants), and the Department of Commerce (via the Economic Development Administration).

Standards and Results

While RLFs take on projects with above-average risk, borrowers are held to standard financial requirements in loan security. Before a loan is issued, a business or prospective business usually supplies the following documentation:

- business plan
- business experience and management information
- credit history and financial statements
- sufficient collateral to repay bank and RLF funding
- other personal or corporate guarantees on the project
- cash flow projections

As a public investment instrument, revolving loan funds are expected to result in public goods—namely projects contributing to economic growth and community revitalization. Borrowers therefore must address performance measures established by the loan administrator such as:

- number and type of jobs created or retained
- increase in tax revenue
- private funding relative to public investment
- benefits to low- and moderate-income citizens, from business ownership to job opportunities

Starting a Revolving Loan Fund

If small businesses in a community have issues accessing conventional financing, public and/or private entities can set up a revolving loan fund. Here are some basic steps for starting an RLF:

1. Research existing RLFs and compile samples of application forms, program guidelines, and other materials.

2. Invite lenders and potential borrowers to participate in the design process.

3. Establish the purpose of the RLF. This should include a needs assessment.

4. Set the eligibility requirements for borrowers.

5. Determine the allowed uses of funds as well as prohibited uses.

6. Set a minimum and maximum amount for the loans.

7. Decide if the loans must be matched by existing equity or other sources of funds.

8. Determine the length of the loan term, which may vary based on the use of the loan. For example, the term for a loan to purchase equipment may be based on the life of the product, while a loan for real estate may have a 15-year term.

9. Establish an application fee, origination fee, and policies regarding closing costs. Define the default and delinquency terms.

10. Decide if the interest rate will be variable or fixed and whether the rate will vary based on the project.

11. Develop the loan application form. Create a short application form or checklist to help borrowers determine if they are eligible.

12. Set up a committee to review loan applications.

13. Determine the administrative duties and staffing needs associated with the program.

14. Promote the RLF and capitalize it with funds from grants and individual donations.

15. Provide loans and technical assistance to borrowers.

Revolving loan funds provide critical financing when credit access is limited, supporting the development and expansion of local businesses and other special initiatives. While a revolving loan fund cannot finance projects on its own, it is an integral part of the small business loan package. Borrowers benefit from flexible and favorable terms, and financial institutions enjoy lower overall risk in supporting small businesses. The results include new jobs, new businesses, and a healthier local economy.

Selecting the Right Tools

Though not all financing programs fall neatly within these practice areas, the toolbox approach is designed to provide a more efficient and effective process for addressing financing needs. The toolbox approach also allows economic development professionals the opportunity to test a variety of strategies on a given project, and to combine programs in order to address financing needs.

Putting development finance tools in place is a comprehensive effort involving bold thinking, innovative planning, considerable strategizing, and a fully supported, cooperative effort from all involved. Agencies that fail to build partnerships and cooperative effort typically fail to implement key aspects of the toolbox for a variety of reasons. Resistance to the toolbox approach will likely exist early in the program planning stages, but once the concept is fully understood, it should be embraced throughout the community.

Keep in mind that not all agencies will manage each of the toolbox elements inside the agency. The toolbox approach brings a myriad of stakeholders to the table providing many different programs. In fact, some of the most successful agencies have partnerships reaching throughout the community to deliver these programs. These partners may exist at the local, county, regional, state, and federal levels and should all be part of the toolbox.

Assembling a Development Finance Team

Within a community myriad resources are available to finance development, but these resources must be coalesced and assembled accordingly. There are three key elements to assembling your local development finance team.

Partnerships

Partnerships are critical in the development finance space. Within a state, region, county, or city, dozens of potential partners exist to support your development finance efforts, each with tools to contribute to your toolkit.

- **Bedrock tools:** state and local bond issues, bond counsel, financial institutions, trustees, nonprofits, bond banks, special purpose authorities, etc.

- **Targeted tools:** special district and taxing authorities, chambers of commerce and business associations, redevelopment authorities, service providers, state and local issues, financial institutions, developers, etc.

- **Investment tools:** financial institutions, local and national allocatees, syndicators, nonprofit Community Development Corporations, developers, seed and venture funds, Opportunity Zone Fund managers, angel investors, housing authorities, federal agencies, etc.

- **Access-to-capital lending tools:** certified development corporations, small business centers, financial institutions, chambers of commerce and business associations, state and federal agencies, development authorities, special taxing authorities, CDFIs, etc.

Expertise

Economic development agencies looking to engage complex financing mechanisms must have the right expertise assembled to ensure success. Development finance is highly technical and requires significant legal, banking, and project development expertise. At a minimum, your development finance team should have expertise in the following areas:

- land assembly, zoning, and planning
- redevelopment process
- underwriting and lending
- credit analysis
- capital attraction and absorption
- loan monitoring, closing, and borrower management
- capital access
- development agreements
- business retention and expansion
- utilities and services
- business development and attraction
- business life cycle
- legal—tax, accounting, incentives, etc.

Coordination

Within a development agency, considerable structure should be in place to help coordinate development finance activities. Recommended practices include:

- **Intake:** Create a simple way to onboard new business opportunities to be able to quickly assess viability. For redevelopment or development projects, have a simple application process upon initial intake. When conducting small business lending, host your application and intake process online to gather preliminary information. Establish protocols for the initial evaluation of an application for funding and set policies that outline the preliminary steps in the funding process.

- **Evaluation:** Create a concise and clear evaluation process for every request for funding. Use loan committees, development authorities, and panels of experts to help vet and evaluate project feasibility. Employ outside experts for feasibility studies and market analyses. Establish clear policies for applicants to follow in the engagement process. Ensure no undue or unethical behavior is conducted to ensure a fair and reasonable evaluation of each project for potential funding.

- **Single point of contact:** For each program (bond, TIF, loan, etc.) establish a single point of contact to shepherd the applicant through the process. In large agencies, you should commit a single person to guide an applicant along in the process. This ensures stability and consistency in program delivery. In smaller agencies, bifurcate this work within staff that have expertise in the assigned lending area. This allows your team to gain knowledge and expertise in one or two financing areas and ensures more reliable oversight.

- **Avoid political influence:** Development finance decisions should be void of political influence. Nothing evokes an emotional response in a community more than the use of complex public financing programs. Ensure that the decision-making process is free of political entanglements so that projects are financed based on merit and analysis and not on political pressure. Elected leaders are an important part of the decision-making process but should be informed and educated along the way. They should be asked to make their decisions based on unbiased input, clear data, and well-established polices for guiding investment.

- **Monitoring:** An overlooked component of the development finance landscape is post-financing monitoring and compliance. Engaging in a financial agreement is a deal-long commitment. The process of financing does not end with project financing and should survive changes to staffing and community priorities. It is critical that your agency establish structured post-closing monitoring and compliance procedures.

Sharing Risk, Credit, and Expenses

An important element of the development finance toolbox is the ability to spread risk and credit and to share the expenses of running programs. Very few development finance agencies are able or willing to accept all of the risk involved in financing business and industry. Even fewer have the financial resources to absorb the operating costs of all of these programs.

Conversely, support agencies, such as Community Development Corporations and port authorities, can play a pivotal role in financing specific development needs and have fee structures that allow them to complete these transactions.

The private sector should also be considered a risk- and credit-sharing partner. The private sector is an eager and willing participant in the development finance toolbox and provides a far greater depth of risk ability than other partners. Private-sector entities such as banks, thrifts, credit unions, syndicators, equity investors, business coalitions, and other private participants all provide opportunities for partnership. In fact, some state and federal laws, such as the Community Reinvestment Act (CRA), mandate that financial institutions make certain amounts of investment in low-income or designated communities. These regulations should be leveraged as part of the process to engage private institutions in the toolbox approach.

The private sector can also address the expenses of running programs, such as revolving loan funds or mezzanine funds. Revolving loan fund banking partners are typically willing to provide loan processing, review, and closing services if partnering loans are banked in their institutions. This provides finance agencies with a great support system and a means to catalyze business financing, while also providing a steady stream of growing businesses—and potential clients—for the banking partner.

Capacity Building and Funding Programs

The natural reaction to the deployment of the toolbox approach is to consider the costs and capacity needed for operating these programs. Understandably, most development agencies and communities do not have the resources to manage all of these efforts. However, the abundance of natural partners within the community, region, and state allows for all of these programs to be deployed at one level or another.

In addition, development finance should be considered a self-sustaining endeavor. The most successful, and often smallest, agencies are able to earn program income from their financing efforts. Take, for instance, a development authority that issues bonds for manufacturers, nonprofits, and other public purposes. This hypothetical agency is able to earn a fee for each transaction up front as well as an ongoing fee through the life of the outstanding bond. These fees typically fund the staffing and compliance aspects needed to manage the program and often allow for greater capacity to serve.

Conversely, take a small nonprofit that manages a revolving loan fund. CDFA estimates that it takes a fund balance of $1.5 million to support one full-time staff person to administer the program. This funding is earned on the entire portfolio of outstanding loans whose borrowers are making regular interest and principal payments (Council of Development Finance Agencies, n.d.). Again, in this example, the portfolio is earning program revenue to support the capacity needed to offer the program.

Build an Adequate Fee Structure

One of the most difficult aspects of the development finance process is the administration and utilization of fees for financing services. Simply put, it costs money to make money, and this holds true in both the public and private sectors. Finance agencies that adhere to a reasonable but strict fee structure for their services are able to provide a higher level of service over agencies that do not require these considerations. The private institutions involved in the bond, tax credit, lending, investment, and other financing programs highlighted in this guide all accept a high level of risk while also accepting a justifiable level of fees for their services. Finance agencies must develop this same mentality and be willing to impose appropriate fees for the use and access to precious public financing resources.

Agencies often struggle with ways to fund these programs; however, the capitalization needed is readily available. A number of funding mechanisms exist:

- **Federal government:** Dozens of federal programs exist to capitalize revolving loan funds and other lending structures.

- **Banks and financial institutions:** These entities have both legal and mission-related requirements for assisting with community development, financial literacy, and access to capital. Hundreds of unique community banking partnerships exist throughout the country, demonstrating the willingness of lending institutions to support development finance. In addition, the federal Community Reinvestment Act (CRA) requires depository institutions to invest in underserved markets. Tools such as CRA are available to build community-banking partnerships and capital for program funding.

- **Foundations:** Philanthropic groups, such as foundations, are playing an increasingly important role in capitalizing development finance programs. These vital partners are active in nearly every state and are willing to support ideas that make a difference. Economic development is a key mission for many of these groups.

- **Industry associations:** Increasingly, industry associations, such as manufacturing and service alliances, are stepping up to support targeted financing programs. These groups wield a strong amount of influence and resources for helping a development agency build programming.

- **Higher education:** Some of the most powerful bonding authorities in the country are universities and colleges. These entities have significant resources for supporting redevelopment, small business, commercialization, and housing.

Communities should engage with these partners to leverage public resources for a win-win outcome.

- **Special assessments:** An increasing number of communities, special districts, and project-specific entities are turning to special assessments to raise capital for development. This mechanism allows businesses, industries, taxpayers, and citizens to opt in to specific projects and programs that cause transformation.

- **Crowdfunding:** Many economic development agencies, nonprofits, small businesses, and entrepreneurs are turning to individual fundraising sources to support capacity building and business development. Crowdfunding is the practice of funding a project or venture by raising monetary contributions from a large number of people. The practice is still in the early stages of development, with state and federal governments currently formulating guidelines and a regulatory framework. This relatively new tool is having a major impact in the development finance industry worldwide.

- **Bond issuance fees:** An often overlooked source of funding for operations and capacity building is bond proceeds. While highly regulated, bond issuers are afforded the authority to apply fees on bond issuances. These can be up-front fees, ongoing annual fees, or a combination of both. The best development agencies effectively use proceeds from bond transactions to fund operations and sustainability.

Public Policy Goals

It is important that the programs in the toolbox adhere to broader public policy goals and that they allocate precious public resources efficiently. By making programs available to businesses and individuals, a development agency is indicating that these tools have been fully vetted, developed, and prepared for use, and that they comply with the guidelines and goals of the agency.

In the field of economic development, the financing of development projects can ultimately impact public policy. When public resources are used to finance projects, the success of these projects is likely to drive future public financing and policy considerations. This is perhaps most critical in urban communities seeking the financial capacity to support redevelopment. By bringing together a variety of parties—including banks, thrifts, educational providers, investors, angels and developers—the toolbox approach may help to expand a community's capacity to take on new economic development projects.

Education is Critical

While it should go without saying, education is the key to building and utilizing the development finance toolbox. The number one reason that agencies cite for not utilizing specific financing tools is a general lack of understanding of a complex tool. Development finance is complex, perhaps overly complex in some instances, and it requires a full understanding from beginning to end to fully employ the variety of tools available. Bonds represent the bedrock financing concepts that have catalyzed a large percentage of the built environment, while newer tools, such as tax credits, have become the primary force driving investment in low-income communities. While both are critical to economic development, one does not outshine the other, and both should be fully understood and utilized.

A variety of training opportunities exist for one to understand the resources available in the development finance toolbox. Organizations such as the national Council of Development Finance Agencies (CDFA at www.cdfa.net) provide training that should be encouraged and enforced by agency leadership. The top agencies in the country dedicate specific resources to building a strong staff with expertise in the toolbox programs.

References

Community Development Financial Institutions Fund. (n.d.). *Opportunity zone resources.* U.S. Department of the Treasury. https://www.cdfifund.gov/opportunity-zones

Council of Development Finance Agencies. (n.d). *Revolving loan fund reference guide.*

Rittner, T. (2009). *Practitioner's guide to economic development finance: Building and utilizing the development finance toolbox.* Council of Development Finance Agencies.

Quality of Place

Talicia Richardson, PCED & Claire Kolberg

Quality of place is defined as the physical characteristics of a community that affect the quality of life of people living and working in it and those visiting it. This chapter will provide participants with an understanding of the role of the arts and culture in community and economic development. By understanding this relationship—and ways to promote engagement at various levels within a community—community developers may achieve outcomes that support quality of place. In addition, strategies in the development of a creative economy as well as potential outputs will be discussed.

Learning Objectives

- Participants will learn how a strong quality of place can promote economic development.

- Participants will understand the role of the arts in civic engagement.

- Participants will learn strategies for supporting a creative economy.

- Participants will learn how the built environment can promote connected, healthy communities.

Quality of place matters. Cultural amenities attract a vibrant workforce, retain families, and build a creative and civic economy. Defined as "the physical characteristics of a community, the way it is planned, designed, developed and maintained that affect the quality of life of people living and working in it and those visiting it both now and in the future" (Burton, 2014), quality of place helps us build the idea that cultural, structural, and economic amenities can boost an community. In short, you can build the kind of city you want to live in.

Importance of Quality of Place

Build it and they will come. What comes first, the chicken or the egg? The expectation with both phrases is that successful execution of quality projects will yield positive outcomes. The incorporation of creative placemaking can encourage attraction to a community regardless of its size (See Case Study *The Unexpected*). The forms of attraction include, but are not limited to, walkable, mixed use environment, increased density through residential living, and diversification in demographics due to an area's physical and social character.

The goal in development and enhancement of cultural amenities is to retain—as well as attract—a qualified workforce while drawing on diverse familial networks that contribute to the building of a creative and civic economy. The expansion of the economy, it is important to note, would include commerce associated with the arts and culture in the form of arts-related businesses and jobs.

Defining Creative Economy

John Howkins, a leading strategist on creativity and innovation, defines creative economy as "economic systems where value is based on imaginative qualities rather than the traditional resources of land, labour and capital. Compared to creative industries, which are limited to specific sectors, the term is used to describe creativity throughout a whole economy" (Farmakis, 2014). While a civic economy is best described as fundamentally both open and social, it is an economy that fuses the culture of web 2.0 with civic purpose (*Compendium for the Civic Economy*, 2011). The National Endowment for the Arts reported that in 2017 "arts and culture added $877.8 billion to the U.S. GDP" (National Endowment for the Arts, 2020).

The arts are an intricate part of society. Since the beginning of time, the use of art was used as a means to communicate. From drawings of prey on cave walls to the piping of music along with wall art placed in a business environment (Alpagu, 2014), the relationship between art, lifestyle, and economics is further confirmed.

Case Study
The Unexpected

In 2015, the nonprofit 64.6 Downtown was established in Fort Smith, Arkansas. The Unexpected was created as its inaugural event to bring urban and contemporary art to the community, culminating in a week-long event in Downtown Fort Smith. The objective of The Unexpected project was to promote, create, and inspire artistic excellence among artists and spectators through professional arts and arts education, music and thought, while driving cultural and economic growth in the community. The event was funded primarily through donations and sponsorships from the private sector—businesses and individuals—as a means to create an investment and buy-in for the development and sustainability of the creative sector.

The 64.6 Downtown Initiative diverged somewhat from the traditional 12-step community development approach (Leinberger, 2005). The nonprofit and private sectors took the lead on early engagement—focusing on, identifying, and securing physical and cultural assets prior to engaging the larger community. This alternative approach supported a clear vision for creating, organizing, curating, and executing the event.

Initially, as a privately funded initiative, the event's objective was to generate momentum and credibility within the community. By garnering civic engagement through a proven, high-quality program, it eventually led to an even more comprehensive plan for the future growth and development of Downtown Fort Smith (64.6 Downtown, 2017; WRT, 2014). The plan was created to reflect the long-term mutual growth objectives for Downtown, as defined by small business owners, area residents, local government leaders, property owners, and other stakeholders. In forging an approach—whether traditional or alternative—leaders should consider several matters:

- **Impact.** The art experience should be welcoming, innovative and groundbreaking. This can be completed through an external curatorial process that gives access to high-quality emerging and established artists who are breaking boundaries and stereotypes when it comes to outdoor and public art concepts. A second layer of impact is created through the local art scene by utilizing painters, artists and artisans, and art students and teachers during production, providing real-world experience and access to artists at varying stages of their careers in a highly contextualized setting.

- **Efficiency.** By keeping the process internal, the event can be executed quickly. However, one must be aware of ordinances or districts that have regulations that require approval.

- **Private Funds.** Using private funds allows the event creative freedom and eliminates the need to "answer" to tax-paying constituents.

Conclusion: Maintaining creative, production, and budgetary control of the event allows for greater freedom of design, decision making, and execution. However, ensuring relationships with the appropriate city and community leaders creates a sense of participation and ownership that ensures the long-term success and need for art in public spaces.

Civic Engagement

It is imperative in community development to engage the community. In a traditional sense, "citizens are engaged when they play a meaningful role in deliberations, discussions, decision making and/or implementation of projects or programs affecting them" (Penn State, n.d.). The National Association of Community Development Extension Professionals (NACDEP) defines the cooperative dynamic of community development as the "participative democracy, sustainable development, rights, equality, economic opportunity and social justice, through the organization, education and empowerment of people within their communities, whether these be of locality, identity or interest, in urban and rural settings" (NACDEP, 2014). In this chapter, we will explore this concept and its role in the arts.

Utilizing public art to drive civic engagement and economic development, while leveling the playing field when it comes to accessing the arts, can promote diversity and inclusion and bestow a unique identity upon a community. When seeking to enhance connectivity between community and economy, it is imperative to develop an all-encompassing master plan. This strategic approach could bring both public and private sectors together for a collaborative plan that is mutually beneficial.

A comprehensive master plan may drill down to a downtown-centric focus and encompass real estate development, arts and culture, job creation, and placemaking, as well as public and private investment decisions through unified planning efforts for smart and sustainable growth (See Case Study *Downtown Connectivity*).

With the engagement of the public sector comes responsibility and accountability. Project leaders should listen attentively in an effort to seek understanding while maintaining the organization's core mission and objectives. This can be one of the most difficult aspects of creating quality of place yet the most rewarding. In developing a master plan for your downtown, consider the following:

- Public gathering spaces: What spaces can be leveraged to make your community unique and desirable for locals—families and individuals—and tourists alike? How can you leverage current cultural activity centers while ensuring growth and sustainability?

- Public infrastructure: How can your downtown be more vibrant, pedestrian friendly, business friendly, and resident friendly?

- Residential properties: How can the community be resident friendly? What access to housing is available, and is there a variety of types of housing to meet folks at different life stages?

- Commercial businesses, restaurants, and entertainment venues: How can dollars be kept local? What daily amenities are needed to fulfill the needs of residents living in downtown, such as groceries and gas?

- Transportation issues: Are there safety concerns or traffic issues that hinder perceptions? Can existing public transportation be utilized differently, expanded, or both?

- Removing obstacles that hinder development: The development process with your city should be recalibrated and streamlined to enable projects to be implemented in a more collaborative and success-driven manner.

Supporting the Creative Economy

The arts community has not been fully realized as an economic driver in most communities; however, there has been an increase in recognition and understanding of the role of the arts within the economy from a creative perspective. The Economic Alliance of Greater Baltimore reports, "The arts are certainly an important part of a strong economy for a number of reasons. In addition to building and amplifying the success of innovative industries, an accessibility to the arts makes a region a more attractive place to live for people and families working in any industry" (Economic Alliance of Greater Baltimore, 2020).

In the development of a creative economy, the connection of community and with community is key in the foundation building phase. E.A. Bucchianeri stated, "Art is in the eye of the beholder, and everyone will have their own interpretation" (Bucchianeri, 2011). Communities must define what strategic moves need to be executed to bring attention to a city as an arts and artist-friendly community while establishing the community as a leader in world-class public art.

A Strong Foundation for Supporting a Creative Economy

To stay relevant, a community may seek to find ways to develop and produce an arts and cultural event for their town. The first step in determining if a large-scale public art event is right for your community is to perform a needs assessment. The following example illustrates recommended steps for conducting a needs assessment specific to your community:

- **Historical significance:** Can a community's historical past coexist with its vibrant future?

  - "This Town USA" is a true western town, established in 1817 as a military post along the western frontier. It played a significant role during the 1830s era of Indian removal, managing thousands of Native Americans entering Indian Territory (modern-day Oklahoma), as well as in-fighting between new and existing tribes in the territory.

  - Gateway to the West: "This Town USA" was the largest federal district in the U.S. at the time, which included Indian Territory.

  - The Eco-Friendly State: "This Town USA" is nestled along a river, once a major artery for transportation and trade, fishing and water access. The area boasts native flora and fauna with unique green space and landscapes still largely untouched by man.

  - Conclusion: The historic past set against modern, contemporary art creates a dynamic juxtaposition. Artists pull from historical and natural references to influence their work, drawing attention to historical and current social and environmental issues.

- **Canvases and infrastructure:** Are there buildings with interesting facades that support mural or other types of art activations? Are there locations that might benefit from an art installation—for example, an empty lot, building, or underused space?

- Does your downtown support an easily walkable experience?

- Underused/underutilized spaces: Are there empty storefronts and a lack of amenities such as coffee shops, retail, and restaurants?

- Civic spaces: How can a partnership with the city, utilizing their spaces, be of benefit to all stakeholders?

- Conclusion: "This Town USA" can support a variety of artistic activations that boast different genres to create a unique art experience. Utilizing relationships with property owners as well as civic leaders allows for ease in securing sites.

- **Purpose:** The key question that guides the decision-making process is, "What is the goal of the event?"

  - Community engagement: Revitalization efforts strengthen a community's existing economic assets while expanding and diversifying its economic base. The event must help in sharpening the competitiveness of existing businesses and new economy used to build a downtown that responds to current consumer needs. Converting unused or underused commercial space into economically productive property also helps to boost the profitability of the community. Additionally, increasing volunteerism and alternative methods of engagement, such as guided art tours and social media engagement, enhances a community's experience.

  - Well-being: Do the activities contribute to a mentally, physically, and economically healthy community? Have perceptions been challenged—not just those that outsiders have of the community but the perceptions the community has of itself—particularly those around social issues, stereotypes, and myths surrounding segments of the community?

  - Sustainability of programs: Can your community capture art space without duplicating what other existing organizations are already doing? Find ways to utilize key partnerships to promote and enhance programs while building awareness of the overall creative economy.

  - Conclusion: "This Town USA" has a sound foundation to begin the works to execute a program to drive engagement, economic growth, and program longevity.

Promotion of Well-Being

With the establishment of the built environment, the community is ripe for further enhancement. As particular areas within a city grow, many downtowns are left with obsolete, underutilized, and vacant buildings as new centers emerge through urban sprawl. This trend suggests that, without action and swift execution of a strategic plan, the existing efforts to revitalize forgotten or failing downtowns or Main Streets could be compromised and contribute to the growing blight and obsolescence in downtown neighborhoods with minimal infill, redevelopment, and adaptive reuse of buildings in older neighborhoods and commercial areas.

Case Study
Universal Chapel to Gateway Park

In 2016 the organizers of The Unexpected invited Spanish artist Okuda San Miguel to complete a 360-degree mural takeover at Rogers and Garrison Avenues, a major intersection into Downtown Fort Smith. The lot was home to a tiny, plain, white office building, shaped like a small house, that had been empty for 25 years. Directly behind the office building was a private park ensconced with a large growth of trees that, while beautiful, was largely ignored by the community with visibility hindered by the empty office and lot.

Upon completion of The Unexpected 2016, Okuda San Miguel transformed the intersection and building into the Universal Chapel, a beautiful painted structure of human sensibility, where all are welcome. The building was embraced by the community, becoming a beacon of positivity and serving as a gateway into Downtown Fort Smith, captivating the community with its powerful color and symbolism. The piece was featured in the most popular trade magazines and blogs including designboom ("Okuda San Miguel," 2019) and was named in *Parade* magazine's "Mural's Across America: The Best Street Art in Every State" in 2019 (Luna, 2019).

In 2017, Unexpected inaugural artist Ana Maria was living in Fort Smith, a result of the deep and meaningful connection she had forged with the community while painting during the first event in 2015. Inspired by the need for arts engagement, Ana Maria opened an art school, La Colmena (The Beehive) in the newly transformed building. 64.6 Downtown offered the space to her rent-free to encourage small business development, with a grow-up plan for rent to activate and increase incrementally as the business grew. The classes were open to all ages and provided an opportunity for arts learning and engagement with a globally renowned working artist.

But with all street art, the Universal Chapel activation was not meant to be a permanent solution. In 2018 the artwork served its purpose when 64.6 Downtown was approached by business and community leaders who envisioned rejuvenating the site into something new—a welcoming entry point into Downtown and a community gathering space complete with educational statues honoring Fort Smith's past, a plaza and green space for gathering and contemplation, that would be gifted by 64.6 Downtown to the City of Fort Smith upon completion.

Through local fundraising and a generous donation by Bancorp South, who owned the park behind the building, Gateway Park was developed. The park includes a plaza with three statues of early Fort Smith community leaders; Judge Isaac Parker, frontier judge and community leader, is the featured subject. He represents law and order in the late 1800s and was an advocate for equal opportunity in education and for women's rights. Judge Parker is joined by John Carnall, who represents public education, and Sister of Mercy, Mother Superior Mary Teresa Farrell, who represents the establishment of healthcare. In October 2019 the park was completed and the deed was transferred from 64.6 Downtown to the City of Fort Smith, completing this public/private partnership.

Influence on Walkability

Public art can reimagine ways people can interact with art and downtown, drawing from the pages of Jeff Speck's *Walkable City* (Speck, 2012) by making a walk intentional and interesting. An outdoor art gallery allows for the intentionality of strategic placement throughout the downtown corridor for various levels of participation. The creation of this outdoor art gallery supports a healthy and connected community. A segment of gallery visitors can opt for the drive-by view via car or bike. With vehicle entry, others stumble onto the experience by simply driving downtown, while others with limited mobility choose to interact with artworks from a vehicle. Pedestrians want to feel safe and comfortable just as much as they would like to be entertained. Public art contributes to the health and wellness of the community by utilizing visuals to promote a walkable downtown (See Case Study *Response to Local Wellness Conditions on Communities*).

Case Study
Response to Local Wellness Conditions on Communities

From 2016 through 2019, the City of Fort Smith prioritized wellness and fitness and spearheaded a fight against pressing health issues. The objectives were formed by the City of Fort Smith Board of Directors in collaboration with various nonprofit organizations, including 64.6 Downtown. These objectives have current and long-term value for the community. They include creating more parks, open space, bike and walking trails, and athletic areas that will be permanent, healthy motivators for the population. The movement aims to increase connectivity and walkability of our city while promoting more natural physical activity within the Fort Smith area.

According to Aspire Arkansas (Smithwick, n.d.), Arkansas ranks 49th in the nation in terms of active adults. In 2017, 33% of adults were not active, up 2 percentage points from 2011 and 7 points higher than the national rate. Sebastian County performs only slightly better than the state average at 29%, while Arkansas state statistics on obesity rates are dismal. The percentage of obese or overweight adults in Arkansas is 70% and rising, while Sebastian County rates are nearly the same at 69%. The need for combative efforts against these issues is dire, and Fort Smith is working to reverse these statistics.

One of the main areas utilized in fulfilling these objectives is the Arkansas Riverfront in Downtown Fort Smith. Projects completed along the Arkansas River include the various artwork installations, the Fort Smith Riverfront Skate & Bike Park, and Greg Smith River Trail. The skate and bike park celebrated its grand opening with more than 1,000 attendees in October 2018. Public and private entities were involved in planning and construction; it is a prime example of the positive outcomes associated with private–public partnerships that target wellness and fitness. The park is a one-of-a-kind attraction that features pump tracks (bike tracks that simulate off-road riding), a 12-foot vertical wall, mountain bike playground, and skating features. Art is integrated into the park, which enables it to simultaneously serve as a place of exercise and inspiration with the Arkansas River as its backdrop.

Walking and biking trails occupy the riverfront, with plans of connectivity to east Fort Smith, which nestles the river. The continued addition of trails in Fort Smith aims to raise the walkability rating of the community from its current walk score of 35 (Walk Score, 2021). The Greg Smith River Trail, known locally as "River Walk," has expanded in three stages since its inception in 2016. The trail runs the western border of the city and river, extending over six miles of paved trailways. In addition to nature sights, there is a stone walkway leading to the Arkansas River for fishing, a pedestrian bridge, pavilion, seating areas, five bronze statues donated by a local family, and artwork installations of *Halite with Quartz and Bauxite* by Paul

Siebenthal and Alex Cogbill along with Brian Massey's *Windsong II*. This picturesque trail begins at the National Historic Site, transitions to the Riverfront Amphitheater along the skate and bike park, passes the U.S. Marshals Museum, and continues to a recently purchased wetland.

The City of Fort Smith has purchased 330 acres of wetland along the Arkansas River. The plan is to create a design that features "multiuse soft service trails for hikers, runners, walkers and cyclists" (Dale, 2018). The walkability rating of the downtown area, where the parks are located, is 58, with a biking score of 56 (Walk Score, 2021).

To further complement cultural amenities through outdoor activities, the increased activation of the Riverfront with its open public access to the Arkansas River, National Historic Site, enhanced multiuse trails, and site of the U.S. Marshals Museum has drawn attention to downtown. As a regional hub for outdoor recreation and a destination rich in local and regional history, awareness of—and the need for—these cultural amenities has grown to maintain a healthy and creative economy.

There are approximately five parks located in Downtown Fort Smith, and 64.6 Downtown has injected two additional green spaces: Garrison Commons and Gateway Park. Garrison Commons pocket park was introduced in 2015, transforming a burned-out lot into an outdoor setting, nestled between two buildings on Main Street with lighting, food truck space, picnic tables, and a small 8x12-foot stage. Garrison Commons transforms into a venue for mixers, corporate events, live music concerts, or private soirees. Gateway Park, dedicated in October 2018, offers a reimagined entrance into Downtown that is a beautifully landscaped park incorporating three statues of figures with historical significance to Fort Smith.

Finally, The Unexpected is an anchor that complements initiatives for health and wellness by augmenting healthy initiatives and the outdoor experience through public art.

While Downtown is the heart and soul of the community, the city is further enhanced by the development of Chaffee Crossing. "The Fort Chaffee Redevelopment Authority (FCRA) and the City of Fort Smith are currently partnering to add an additional 6.5 miles of trails to connect all of Chaffee Crossing to the Fort Smith Master Trail Plan and regional trails" ("Outdoor recreation," n.d.). The walkability of the Massard neighborhood, which is the closest rated area to Chaffee Crossing, is 39. It is the third most walkable neighborhood in Fort Smith (Walk Score, 2021). Money for the trails will come from a city 1/8% sales tax for parks, which the city Finance Department estimates generates more than $2.6 million a year. The FCRA has also pledged $500,000 toward development of each of the three segments of the project. A $500,000 Transportation Alternatives Program grant from the Arkansas Department of Transportation will help pay for the first segment.

The second segment of the project, which the Fort Smith Parks and Recreation Department estimates will cost $750,000, consists of extending the first segment from McClure Drive southwest about a mile to Massard Road near the Wells Lake Road intersection. Work on the second was completed in the spring of 2021. A parks department capital improvement plan puts the cost of the segment at $2.1 million. The FCRA is mindful of incorporating walkable designs that naturally promote physical activity into its infrastructure development.

Throughout Downtown and Chaffee Crossing, 64.6 Downtown and FCRA strives to bridge the connectivity of Fort Smith from west to east with the support of the City of Fort Smith. The efforts described have been largely successful and supported by the community. The skate and bike park is a popular designation with younger residents, and the Greg Smith River Trail sees traffic from approximately 100 individuals each day as reported by the Metropolitan Planning Organization (TRAFx Research, n.d.).

Although developed for Fort Smith, these projects are scalable in any community that desires to promote health and outdoor activities. Partners involved in the previously mentioned projects included the City of Fort Smith Administration and Parks & Recreation, private donors, Friends of Recreational Trails, 64.6 Downtown, Fort Chaffee Redevelopment Authority, Western Arkansas Planning & Development District, and the citizens of Fort Smith. These partnerships provided funding, volunteers, staff support, and in-kind donations.

Case Study
Downtown Connectivity

Downtown Fort Smith's mobility network is unique when compared to other traditional historic downtowns in the region. The robust commercial corridor of Garrison Avenue serves as the Main Street, instead of a traditional courthouse square or plaza with historic buildings around all sides. Fort Smith has several unique districts and neighborhoods that make up its downtown core, each accentuated and enhanced by pockets of historic architecture and buildings.

Fort Smith is also fortunate to have access to all modes of transportation including air, rail, road, and water. However, due to its proximity to interstate highways and the Arkansas River, many of the roadways in the Central Business Improvement District (CBID) radiate from Downtown, providing a convenient cut-through for cars and trucks seeking a quicker alternative across the river.

This transportation-focused framework has also led to Downtown's fragmentation and perception of a lack of connectivity and safety as development became more auto-centric. What was once a bustling corridor with horses, carriages, trolleys, and wide pedestrian realms has transformed into a significant regional transit corridor. This has also impacted the type of development that has come into the area and left many of the neighborhoods disconnected or less walkable.

An initial mobility analysis identified key economic corridors in the CBID (64.6 Downtown, 2017). This analysis was done in coordination with the catalytic development opportunities identified in the plan and through the public feedback received during the early engagement process. This early evaluation also included looking at the existing corridor characteristics, focusing on the following:

- available street right-of-way
- existing lane configurations
- recent traffic volumes
- condition of existing facilities
- surrounding land uses
- presence of pedestrian sidewalks, bicycle facilities, transit routes
- future planned capital improvements

The downtown transportation system is now challenged with finding a balance between accommodating the current demand for regional commerce versus serving local trip-making for residents and merchants. (64.6 Downtown, 2017).

Conclusion

Quality-of-place creation should be a goal for which all communities strive. The utilization of arts and culture in the development of such a place is proven to provide a holistic economy while bringing civic engagement into the fold. Continuous assessment of community needs, including quality execution of a strategic plan, will support a sustainable creative economy.

About 64.6 Downtown

64.6 Downtown was created to act as a catalyst for economic development in Downtown Fort Smith by inspiring and engaging partners through art and arts education, placemaking, and other attractive amenities, as a means to accelerate development of diverse commerce. 64.6 represents the square miles of the City of Fort Smith when the organization was founded by entrepreneur and businessman Steve Clark.

Initiatives of 64.6 Downtown include: Garrison Commons pocket park, Gateway

Park, Propelling Downtown Forward Master Plan, and the inaugural event of 64.6 Downtown, The Unexpected.

The Unexpected was founded in 2015, bringing urban and contemporary art, music, speakers, and art education opportunities to Arkansas, culminating in a week-long event in Downtown Fort Smith.

References

64.6 Downtown. (2017, July). *Propelling Downtown forward*. https://www.646downtown.com/projects. https://8b802728-bc53-4aff-bfb6-0692cf248063.filesusr.com/ugd/5ad716_1233890533484e43b182b35b6d9b43e7.pdf

Alpagu, H. (2014). Economy and art: Why are economy and art closely linked? *Journal of Economics Library, 1*(1) http://www.kspjournals.org/index.php/JEL/article/view/158

Bucchianeri, E.A. (2011). *Brushstrokes of a gadfly*. Batalha Publishers

Burton M. (2014) Quality of place. In A.C. Michalos. (Ed.) *Encyclopedia of Quality of Life and Well-Being Research*. Springer. https://doi.org/10.1007/978-94-007-0753-5_2381

Compendium for the civic economy: What the Big Society should learn from 25 trailblazers. (2011). https://issuu.com/architecture00/docs/compendium_for_the_civic_economy_publ

Dale, T.A. (2018, November 13). *Fort Smith may acquire 330 acres near downtown for trails*. Talk Business & Politics. https://talkbusiness.net/2018/11/fort-smith-may-acquire-330-acres-near-downtown-for-trails/

Economic Alliance of Greater Baltimore. (2020). *The importance of the arts in economic development*. www.greaterbaltimore.org/news/blog/importance-arts-economic-development

Farmakis, E. (2014, November 24). Fostering the creative economy. *Stanford Social Innovation Review*. https://ssir.org/articles/entry/fostering_the_creative_economy

Leinberger, C.B. (2005, March). *Turning around downtown: Twelve steps to revitalization*. Brookings. https://www.brookings.edu/research/turning-around-downtown-twelve-steps-to-revitalization/

Luna, K. (2019, July 26). *Murals across America: The very best street art in every state*. Parade. https://parade.com/899760/kristinluna/best-murals-street-art-every-state/#gallery_899760-4

National Association of Community Development Extension Professionals (NACDEP). (2014). *What is community development?* (2014). https://www.nacdep.net/what-is-community-development-

National Endowment for the Arts. (2020, March). *The U.S. arts economy (1998–2017): A national summary report.* https://www.arts.gov/sites/default/files/The-US-Arts-Economy-(1998%E2%80%902017)-A-National-Summary-Report.pdf

Okuda San Miguel turns an abandoned house in Arkansas into a "universal chapel." (2019, December 12). designboom | architecture & design magazine. https://www.designboom.com/art/okuda-san-miguel-universal-chapel-justkids-arkansas-09-20-2016/

Outdoor recreation. (n.d.). Fort Chaffee Redevelopment Authority. http://www.chaffeecrossing.com/amenitiesrecreation/outdoor-recreation

Penn State College of Agricultural Sciences. (n.d.) *Why Community Engagement Matters.* https://aese.psu.edu/research/centers/cecd/engagement-toolbox/engagement/why-community-engagement-matters

Smithwick, K. *Health.* (n.d.). Aspire Arkansas. https://www.aspirearkansas.org/health

Speck, J. (2012). *Walkable city: How downtown can save America, one step at a time.* Farrar, Straus and Giroux.

TRAFx Research: Vehicle counter, trail counter, bike counter. (n.d.). https://www.trafx.net

Walk Score. (2021). *Fort Smith neighborhoods.* https://www.walkscore.com/AR/Fort_Smith

WRT for the City of Fort Smith. (2014, December). *Future Fort Smith; A comprehensive plan for the City of Fort Smith, Arkansas.* http://www.fortsmithar.gov/index.php/future-fortsmith. https://www.fortsmithar.gov/index.php/future-fortsmith

YEAR III

Community Leadership Development
Rhonda L. McClellan

Marketing Your Community
Amanda Sutt & Valerie Kinney

Measuring Community Progress
Rhonda Phillips

Workforce Planning and Development
Courtney Taylor & Heather Annulis

Community Leadership Development

Rhonda L. McClellan, EdD

This session will explore how through self-reflection, community leaders can be more self-aware and hence clearer about how they orient towards leadership. Leader orientation is informed by social convention, context, and private aspirations. Conventional approaches to leadership often enable the status quo. In today's context, however, our communities face volatility, uncertainty, complexity, and ambiguity (VUCA), a new norm. Private aspirations about how to lead in such a context must confront conventional approaches and sense how to adapt leadership approaches. Dialogic, agile, and inclusive leadership sustains resilient communities in the VUCA context.

Learning Outcomes

- Participants will learn how to self-reflect upon and self-regulate their leader identities.

- Participants will learn how to identify the difference between leader-centric and collective approaches to leadership and indicate their own preferences.

- Participants will learn how to recognize and navigate complexity.

- Participants will learn how to execute aspects of cogenerative dialogue.

- Participants will learn how to adopt agile approaches to leadership.

- Participants will learn how to include diverse social capital and cultivate respect and empathy.

- Participants will learn how to lead during times of uncertainty and/or crisis.

> The true mark of a leader is the willingness to stick with a bold course of action—an unconventional business strategy, a unique product-development road map, a controversial marketing campaign—even as the rest of the world wonders why you're not marching in step with the status quo. In other words, real leaders are happy to zig while others zag. They understand that in an era of hyper-competition and nonstop disruption, the only way to stand out from the crowd is to stand for something special.
>
> —Bill Taylor, former U.S. ambassador (2010)

Community leaders confront a shifting social milieu. Who would question that terrorism, social unrest, economic meltdowns, climate change, and pandemics have cultivated a world of turbulence and crises? Most scholarship about the VUCA (Volatile, Uncertain, Complex, and Ambiguous) context prompts leaders to "voluntarily engage in fear" (Johansen, 2017, p. 39), heal fragmented relationships, harvest the riches of our diverse communities (Brown, Harris & Russell, 2010), and "shape our interior response" (Scharmer, 2016, p. 243). Leaders are "to create a space for cosensing what is going on, a space for letting go of the old and cocreating the new" (Scharmer, 2016, p. 243). To hone a leader identity fit for such a context, today's community developers go on an inward journey, first acknowledging conventional expectations of leadership and then adapting to and disrupting those expectations. They must sense the VUCA context and bravely lean into its future.

As a developing leader, you should be prepared for challenges. Your inward journey could further assist in exposing how your assumptions about and preferences for a particular type of leadership and the leader you aspire to become orient you toward a particular leader identity. Your leadership orientation—either implicitly or explicitly—can be captured by a leadership platform, a "bottom-line reminder of what is ethical and valuable" (Ivory, 2015, p. 15). Whereas a leadership platform will keep you situated as you make decisions and move through quandaries, experiences and contexts can shift and evolve. Your platform and your identity can be questioned and developed. Leaders within the VUCA context learn what Scharmer (2016) prompts to "become aware and change the *inner space* from which we operate" (p. 10).

Leadership approaches have historically been understood as either the conventional and egocentric or the emergent and collective. When situations become destabilized, unpredictable, and complex—when racial tension, pandemics, climate change, economic disenfranchisement, disruptive technologies, and political paralysis and dysfunction spiral our communities into chaos—leadership platforms must transform and emerge into the future.

For communities to be sustainable and resilient in the VUCA context, leadership must extend even beyond the collective approach. People today who have accepted the mantle of leadership do so at a transitional time in history. Most of any modeling and training they have received is insufficient for the VUCA context. To be fit for this context, they must transform the leader they have yet to become and scholarship has yet to prescribe. They must learn with new mental models, sense into the future, maneuver with agility, and cocreate knowledge within the larger system.

The Makings of a Leader

Leaders are guided by their values and beliefs. Often. though. leaders resist the reflective practice of accounting for their leadership expectations. If they were to consider why leaders matter and what their contributions should be, they might arrive at a deeper self-awareness of who they aspire to become and the ways in which they should chart their own growth. They would arrive at a vision for their leader identity. Your leadership platform—leadership preferences and models, values, and definitions—align with leadership approaches. Crafting your own can be an important first step in uncovering your beliefs and values about leadership.

Much of what leaders believe about leadership derives from their experiences and observations of leadership. Leaders remember individuals who modeled good and bad leadership. If experience allows, good leaders exemplify the principles of exemplary leadership. They clearly (a) expressed and modeled their values, (b) inspired a shared vision by incorporating common values, challenged status quo, and encouraged innovation, (c) supported collaboration and facilitated professional relationships, and (d) demonstrated appreciation for people by contributing to their development (Kouzes & Posner, 2017). Sometimes experience provides encounters with poor leadership, models developing leaders attempt to avoid. These role models substantiate perceptions of and preferences for particular leadership approaches. They become a part of a leader's repertoire and are all rooted in the past. Leadership expectations are built upon on historical and conventional examples.

> **Modeled Leadership Practice**
>
> Developing a leader identity is contingent, in part, upon self-reflection and self-awareness. Becoming more aware of who you aspire to be as a leader comes with reflecting about your values and beliefs about leadership. Take the time to consider and write a response to the following questions:
>
> - Why are leaders important to their communities?
> - How do leaders function within them, and why are they needed?
> - What is the outcome of ideal leadership?
> - How does a leader use their influence?
> - How does a leader use their power?

Leader Attributes

Besides exemplary behaviors, people perceive and respond to particular leadership attributes. These implicit preferences are subject to context and have the power to establish accepted leadership prototypes (Offermann & Coats, 2018). People believe that leaders should have traits and behaviors they are familiar with. Because they are familiar with these attributes, people prefer, value, and emulate them; such attributes are reinforced by familiarity, observation, and practice. Preferred leader attributes are difficult but not impossible to shift.

Acknowledging implicit biases toward certain kinds of leaders and leadership behaviors can call into question who is allowed to lead and what is considered exemplary leadership. Attributes found to be prototypical of leaders include: sensitive, dedicated, in control, charismatic, strong, creative, well-groomed, masculine, and intelligent (Offermann & Coats, 2018). As Offermann and Coats found, implicit leadership trait bias can perpetuate preferred leader attributes. For developing leaders, the search for authenticity should be troubled. If leader identities are influenced by previous leaders who modeled conventional leadership behaviors and represented preferred leader attributes and prototypes, how much of a leader identity is situated in the authentic self? And how much of that identity has been handed down by those historically in power? How willing have leaders been able to let go of the "old self"? How willing have they been to zag when others zig?

Modeled Leadership Practice

For this reflective activity, list 15 preferred traits that you value in leaders. Narrow the list down to your top three traits. From this narrowed list, think of a leader you admire or admired who modeled one of these three attributes. Then, write a description of this leader's behaviors and traits.

What did this leader embody, and why did you admire them? When you think of the leaders who have influenced your own leader identity, what attributes and behaviors come to mind? What did they model and what of your own identity emulates what you observed?

Reflect upon the ways in which their leadership has influenced your own leader identity. Explore how you are becoming like them and how you are different or strive to be different from them despite your admiration.

Leader Values

Values are inherent in every critical decision leaders make, and the "clearer [they] are about [their] values, the easier it is for them and everyone to commit to the chosen path and stay on it" (Kouzes & Posner, 2017, p. 55). Kouzes and Posner also note that leaders must set the example by aligning their actions with shared values. This means that leaders should (1) spend time on things that matter, (2) watch their language, (3) ask purposeful questions, (4) and seek feedback (pp. 75–85). Values are derived from beliefs and convictions.

How much conviction a leader has toward a particular value, however, will not be realized until it is tested. A leader will encounter conflict between espoused values, and the prioritization of them will be clearer once tested. These encounters are known as *critical incidents*. Knowing their personal histories before attending to the present and prospecting the future can provide leaders guidance and inform their choices. Researchers have noted that leaders should learn to narrate critical incidents. Weaving their values and critical incidents through storytelling conveys to others and reminds themselves as to what is valued. Members, in turn, judge these life stories as a leader's authenticity (Shamir & Eilam, 2005). Storytelling and capturing critical events to convey values assist leaders in leader identity development.

Storytelling and Values Practice

Developing your point of view and values from personal experiences, personal reflection, and personal learning is essential to leader development and your leadership platform. Identifying critical events and telling stories about those events can convey to others your value system and point of view. Followers will judge your authenticity by the stories you tell and their concordance with your espoused values.

If you were to identify three episodes in your past that still resonate with you today, what would they be? Be able to draw upon each of these events and draw out in a narrative what happened and why you believe it was important. Reflect upon how it cultivated who you are and what you believe. Note how your belief conveys what you value.

As a leader, have such narratives tucked away, ready for conveying to others when you want to portray your values—not only for storytelling, but for reminding yourself what you value and why you do. Your values become the cornerstone of your leadership identity and platform. Write a narrative for the critical incidents of your life. Then add a section that explains why the event was important to you. Identify what you learned from the event and why it resonates with you today. Explain how it represents one of your values.

Leadership Approaches

> 2020 has been a banner year. As we navigate the current pandemic crisis in our various municipalities, leadership and sound decision making becomes key to keeping our citizens safe and our communities functioning. The challenges have been unique with no clear answers or guidance in some circumstances. Normal decision-making processes have had to be retooled to take into consideration the unknown effects of the virus and the need to still provide essential services—in a safe and responsible way. I personally have had to make decisions that affect the lives of hundreds, while balancing the various levels of concern for city worker safety, resident well-being, and business leaders whose bottom line is affected by my decisions.
>
> —E. Dunbar, Mayor (personal communication, 2020)

Leadership identities are also informed by the way leaders themselves define leadership. Leadership definitions typically consider people, influence, and movement. But arriving at one agreed-upon definition has proven difficult. Many of these definitions describe one person directing or motivating others to fulfill vision and carry out outcomes. These descriptions place the leader in the center of the action of the organization, a puppet master pulling strings so that they can have their way. This leader is perceived as being a complete leader, someone who has all the necessary intelligence, expertise, and skills needed to fix all problems and maintain order within the community. In slightly different descriptions this puppet master is more benevolent—a therapist, a savior, or an innovator who learns how to motivate others so they can accomplish the leader's goals.

Defining leadership is often embedded into the way the leader approaches it. Approaches are generally divided into two categories: *leader-centric* and *collective*.

Leader-centric approach: The leader-centric approach places the leader in official positions of authority and at the top of organizational structure. This conventional view of leadership promotes change as a way to fix problems through planned, strategic stages; disequilibrium must be temporary and returned to stasis as quickly as possible. Conflict, disruption, or differing opinions are results of flawed management. Teams and relationships are organized and used by the leader to fulfill projects and plans. According to these descriptions, effective leaders should be intelligent, decisive, directing, extraverted/social, and dependable.

Leader-centric approaches have been framed by a variety of leadership theories. Trait theories focused on the individual's attributes. Early theories in this area believed leaders were born with specific traits, such as intelligence, height, extraversion, openness, or narcissism. Scholars would identify the Big Five: intellect, dependability, surgency, agreeableness, and emotional stability (Judge, Bono, Ilies & Gerhardt, 2002). It was argued that leader traits remained constant over time and across situations. Such constraints could not produce predictors of leadership effectiveness or explain why they were important, so the area of study lost attention.

Other leader-centric theories included behavioral, situational, leader-member exchanges, transactional, transformational, charismatic, and authentic (Stone & Patterson, 2005). Behavioral theories focused on the leader's styles: task-orientation vs. people-orientation, authoritarian, pacesetter, democratic, or laissez-faire. Scholars noted that leaders' orientations toward people or tasks altered the way they interacted with people. Out of this school of thought, situational leadership theorists noted that if leaders intentionally changed their behavior given the follower's needs and the task at hand, they could motivate followers to comply and perform. Scholars began to acknowledge leadership was also contingent upon leaders, a dyadic relationship between leader and follower and, later, among leader and the collective communities. In organizations, power, influence, and decision making were isolated by and granted to a few key players who could find simple explanations about how to solve the problem. Leaders fixed problems and righted the world.

Collective leadership approach: For community leaders, however, organizational bureaucracies and hierarchies and management of people through "command and compliance" (Schweigert, 2007, p. 326) does not account for the responsibility of leading for the common good in a shared-power world (Crosby & Bryson, 2005). Imagine being a single parent, working an essential job during a pandemic, while your child is left at home to be schooled virtually. Imagine being a university professor of environmental science who witnesses city employees pouring herbicides and pesticides along the city trail and creek system. Imagine being a man experiencing homelessness and being dependent upon the local ministry for shelter. Imagine the many people being represented by your leadership and your commitment to them. And remember, all residents have a voice and vote in community leadership. Community leadership is both collective and emergent.

Collective leadership focuses on the interconnections and interdependence of all members. Collective leaders humbly admit that they are incomplete and behave like hosts. They invite and host networks to pool resources and integrate their leadership. They operate within flattened hierarchies where decision making occurs throughout the community. Leaders distribute power and authority throughout the organization, making space for self-forming teams and leadership, individuals stepping forward into and falling back out of leadership responsibilities. They value relationships and collaboration. Rather than the act of a single individual in charge of mobilizing others, leadership is a collective action where all residents, through shared power, collaboration, and relationships, participate in leadership for the common good.

Collective leadership approaches are also framed by leadership theories. Cross-sector collaboration (Crosby & Bryson, 2005), integrative leadership (Bono, Shen & Snyder, 2010), and distributed leadership (Bolden, 2011) offer a transition between leader-centric and collective theories. These theories pose that leadership has both administrative-directed and democratically shared power aspects (Bolden, 2011). Social network theory (Cullen-Lester & Yammarino, 2016), complexity leadership (Uhl-Bein & Marion, 2009) and constructionist collective leadership (Endres & Weibler, 2017) offer an emergent, interactive process, cultivating group members' capacity and adaptability through networks and systems. Given that collective leadership is a more recent approach to leadership, several other frames and models are being developed.

Leader-centric and collective leadership approaches describe leadership falling into two general categories. Some focus on leadership as a role and define it as "the ability to get participants in an organization to focus their attention and efforts on the problems that the leader considers significant" (Cyert, 1990). Others propose that leadership is a behavior that emerges within a context of ongoing interactions among individuals and groups "manifest[ing] across different people depending on the nature of interactions" (Plowman & Duchon, 2008, p. 131). Definitions of leadership are embedded within assumptions about control, power, and certainty.

Defining Leadership Practice

You have explored leadership perceptions, preferences, values, and the conceptualizations above. How do you weigh the importance of certainty, control, and power? Do you think it is necessary to have a formal leader, or can leadership be shared among a collective? How would you define leadership for your leadership platform? Let's explore your preferences here.

Before composing your leadership definitions, answer the following questions. On a scale from 1 to 5—1 being "not at all" and 5 being "to the greatest degree"—rate the following:

1. **To what degree is the world knowable?**
    1   2   3   4   5

2. **To what degree can a leader control and predict the direction of their communities?**
    1   2   3   4   5

3. **To what degree can individuals in formal positions of authority own decision-making?**
    1   2   3   4   5

4. **To what degree do leaders influence followers to achieve an outcome?**
    1   2   3   4   5

5. **To what degree should a leader focus on solving problems?**
    1   2   3   4   5

6. **To what degree are leaders found within formal positions of authority?**
    1   2   3   4   5

7. **To what degree can supervisors influence followers to achieve an outcome?**
    1   2   3   4   5

8. **To what degree should leaders engage others in addressing challenges?**
    1   2   3   4   5

Navigating VUCA Context and Turbulence

The many challenges that communities face today create an environment of instability and constant change. These challenges require innovative leaders who can create a positive impact within their community through change initiatives and collaboration to develop opportunities for both individuals and businesses within those communities. Successful community leaders recognize, encourage, and support community participants during these turbulent times. Offering professional development activities, engaging participants in decision making, and creating a support network are some ways positive impact occurs in a community.

—L. Jackson, County Leadership Development Officer and business owner (personal communication, June 2020)

Community leaders must navigate in communities where deeply held beliefs and values that once united and promoted communities become less relevant and more divisive. It's no secret community leaders must confront a multitude of divides. Millions of people face food insecurities, health disparities, low education access, poor technological infrastructure, environmental injustices, and distraught economies. Quality of life is poor for many residents. To build resilient communities, leaders must seek solutions to adaptive challenges. These solutions reside not just within formal positions of authority but also within the "collective intelligence of employees at all levels who need to use one another as resources, often across boundaries, and learn their way to those solutions" (Heifetz & Laurie, 2001, p. 124).

Navigating the VUCA context and the current state of turbulence require community leaders to escape the me/you and us/them structures. Community leadership is now dependent upon the interconnected and interdependent aspects of an ecosystem—environmental, cultural, creative, health, educational, social, and economic. To sustain this ecosystem, leaders must navigate turbulence while being open-minded, open-hearted, and openly willed. They sense the system, their own presence within it, community need, and relationships. Because this leadership is collective and emergent, leaders must be sensing, agile, and inclusive.

Sustaining Resilient Communities

The turbulence we are witnessing in our nation's cities is a symptom of something beyond systemic racism, lack of social or economic justice, or political division. In my opinion it is a symptom of a self-centered and isolated existence which has crippled social development for thousands of years. Positive social change begins with our ability as leaders to think, feel, listen, speak and act with the understanding that it is not about us—it is about the generations which will follow. The decisions we face as leaders must be framed in the context of the future lives of others' children, grandchildren and even great grandchildren, not simply the lives of those we serve today. Placement of constituents' wants or political beliefs ahead of how society should function for all fifty years in the future, is self-serving and should not be considered leadership. As leaders look into the faces of those who are currently impacted by the systemic racism and lack of social or economic justice, we must see the faces of their grandchildren and feel how their lives will be impacted without change. Creating this change must be our motivation—our passion as leaders. Our ability to reflect this in our communities may not create immediate change, but it does reflect compassion and hope to those who are suffering. To live above ourselves and our own interests is the beginning of transformative change for our society. If we who are in public service fail to place others ahead of ourselves how can we expect society to ever change? Leadership is not a job—it is a manner of living and giving, no matter the obstacles encountered.

—Craig Lindholm, City Manager (personal communication, 2020)

As explored in this chapter, leadership identity is critical in the leader development process. When an individual reflects upon their leadership perceptions, preferences, values, and approaches to leadership, they orient their own identity toward leading. In the process of considering what they believe, leaders should also question why they orient in the direction that they do. This self-awareness uncovers implicit biases created by preferred leader prototypes, critical incidents, and encounters with previous leaders. Leaders must sift through the ways in which they have been programmed to lead and their own leadership authenticity. When identities are tested, individuals can hide, protect, or defend; they do nearly anything to preserve sense of self. Their leader identity is contingent upon their ability to define and, most importantly, to redefine leadership within a new context. Leaders must be able to make meaning for themselves and have the strength to "form, repair, maintain, revise their constructions of what it means to lead" (Alvesson & Willmott, 2002, p. 626; Ibarra, 1999). They must self-explore: *If I am a leader, then who am I really?* And, they must be open to pursuing a new self and other new ways of leading. In the VUCA context, leaders may put their old identities on the line in order to become someone new and go about their work differently.

Leaders in times of turbulence notice that doing what was right before does not necessarily produce the results it once had. If leaders allow their well-being to rest on the assumption that they can predict responses, they will feel inept. When their leadership falls short, they will work harder, try to control harder. They may begin to acknowledge that they can control little within a system. If they begin to acknowledge that they are struggling, turn to seek simplicity, and admit they may not achieve solutions, they move closer to acceptance of complexity itself. Accepting complexity makes working within it more palatable and manageable. Expanding the leader identity includes recognizing the seven elements of complexity:

- **Stasis:** This element assumes that the future is fundamentally an extension of the present. Leaders can respond with overconfidence in assuming so.

- **Emergence:** Identities and actions emerge within the system. They are results of previous conditions and causalities in the system. Leaders can begin to shape responses and conditions to the emergence.

- **Feedback loops:** Feedback loops result when a change in one system has secondary effects. Feedback loops can dilute change or feed a virtuous or vicious cycle.

- **Disruptors:** Coming from within or external to the system, disruptors, a form of emergence, perturb the system.

- **Organizing principles:** These are the broad conditions that can assist with the integration or avoidance of complexity. These principles include connectivity, fluidity, or stability. Principles can also offer future direction.

- **Polarities:** These dynamics occur when organizing principles or core beliefs oppose each other, both being important to the community's resiliency.

- **Stillness:** Stillness is experienced as places of pause within communities before decisions are made (Silsbee, 2018, p. 92–100).

Accepting complexity and its elements can lead to deeper self-awareness and self-regulation. When leaders sense complexity, their leadership changes. Part of leader self-awareness is learning to acknowledge and question the leader platform. Systems and identity share many of the elements of complexity. Stasis can stunt identity growth, and emergence can shape it. Feedback can sustain either good or bad character dispositions. Individuals can hold opposing values internally. They must grapple with uncertainty and unclear direction. To navigate such leader identity development, leaders acquaint themselves with learning how to focus and self-regulate through meditative practice and an observing mind. This internal journey provides leaders a sense of the self.

Sensing substantiates a leader identity. Through the sensing process, leaders reflect upon or are confronted by their assumptions, triggers, and aversions. Through self-reflection and purposeful stillness, the observing mind allows leaders to suspend prejudgments and pay attention to the unexamined beliefs they or others have constructed. Sensing allows leaders to be present in complexity, and most importantly, sensing leaders are fully present in relationships. Their mindset becomes open to opposition and diversity; their reactions are less judgmental and assumptive. Their leadership becomes inclusive of others' power and expertise. They suspend their thinking and responses so they can be present in a relationship. Sensing changes leadership, and to lead resilience, community leaders sense VUCA change.

Practice: Sensing the Leadership Mindset

Changing the way we see relationships begins with the way in which we see people. Reflect upon a time when you prejudged an individual. Perhaps you had only part of the information, and with that partial information you came to the wrong conclusion about that individual. Consider these questions:

- How did you learn the truth?
- How did that make you feel?
- How did it do damage to your relationship with that individual?
- How did your prejudgment jeopardize your leadership?
- What if you had stilled your mind and opened it to a different conclusion, one based on more information and without assumptions?

Sensing leaders create new mental models so they do not protect their own interests. They disrupt their own pre-established mental models and embrace new ways of learning. They do not rely only on self-reflection to lead. Leaders of resilient communities acknowledge they alone do not know the answers. They must shift from a leader-centric approach to a collective one in order to lead. They pause and listen to the unfolding future.

Relationships become essential. Leaning into the future, leaders rely upon the collective leadership to cocreate their future. To penetrate deeply into the larger whole, the collective leadership zooms out and hones its capacity for deeper self-awareness and into the broader community (Senge, Scharmer, et al., 2014). Leaders learn to let go of preconceptions, assumptions, the need to control, and of old identities, and a future into the complexity comes through humble inquiry and deep listening.

Humble inquiry and generative listening simplify and clarify the leader's mindset. They sense by receiving energy and information (Silsbee, 2018). Schein (2013) tells us that we learn about culture not by participating but by being conscious and present—by suspending judgmental interactions and respecting the community as a living organism. This communication approach is rooted in mindfulness, similar to meditation, and produces cocreation and cogenerative opportunities. Humble inquiry draws people out by asking sincere questions to learn more about them, building a relationship on curiosity and interest (Schein, 2013). Schein points out that teamwork is like a seesaw with everyone doing their part. For this to occur, leaders foster positive, trusting relationships among members who engage in open conversations. He furthers that leaders should do three things: (1) do less telling, (2) ask more humble and candid questions for the purpose of getting to know people better, and (3) hear and acknowledge that they understand what the person is expressing. The state of listening can be generative, but it requires intentionality from all leaders. Generative listening cannot be forced, but leaders can generate conditions for it. When conversing, leaders should do nothing. They should suspend themselves—in thinking and speaking. They should "stay with and hold the space for what wants to emerge" (Scharmer, 2018, p. 42). This type of inquiry and dialogue generates collective leadership. Through cocreating dialogue, people inquire and listen, and they begin to think and feel together. When this type of dialogue occurs, leaders pay attention to the united silence.

Practice: Cocreating Dialogue

Let's practice cocreating dialogue. Before attending a meeting, make a list of questions that will sincerely open up the flow of information and energy. Ask questions that seek out information you do not know the answer to. Ask questions that will draw out the expertise and experience of others.

Note how the flow of the meeting and the exchange between members shifts. Watch the collaboration. Who is talking? Who is listening? How does asking questions shift the flow of power? Be quiet. Calm your mind. Focus on your breathing: in and out—slowly, deeply. Listen. Hear the collaboration. Wait for the sincere question. Ask the sincere question. Note authenticity.

When you return to your office or car, take a few minutes to reflect upon your humble inquiry and your deep listening. How did cocreating dialogue prolong and deepen collaboration?

Agile Leadership

Agility can occur at the individual, relational, and system levels. It looks distinct from traditional performance. Traditional practice involves 10-year strategic plans, a long-term review process, and formal leaders responsible for executing the plan. Agile practices are people-oriented, self-organizing, and cross-functional (Birkinshaw, 2018). Agile leaders have a deep sense of purpose, clarity, and the ability to switch swiftly from one deep focus to another. They value enablers and disruptors and are connected—to people, the system, and the way into the future. Leaders have transparent, trusting, and positive relationships with people throughout the community. They actively devolve decision making to those closest to the circumstances. They encourage people empathetically and trustingly collaborate throughout the community to achieve shared outcomes and eliminate silos and boundaries. Agile leaders refuse to see things as others do. They disrupt the status quo to create new possibilities, engaging others to make it a reality.

Leaders can develop their agility "muscle" through exercise. Leaders' mental agility can be better developed with meditative states. Taking the time to meditate daily has proven to develop leaders' cognitive abilities to focus and shift. Agility is gathering new tools, competencies, and coping mechanisms (Baran & Woznyj, 2019). Agility is "being at the edge of new knowledge" (Johansen, 2017, p. 137) and is at the heart of resilience. Agile leaders are edgy enough to continuously push their learning to the next stage, always asking themselves the tough questions. They do so to better position themselves for uncertainty, ambiguity, and for sensing out the future. Agile leader lean into the future. Agile leaders draw upon the following practices when addressing community disruption:

- **Communicate:** sharing information bottom up, providing unique perspectives regarding the issue

- **Cogenerate knowledge:** sharing knowledge among cross-functional teams to broaden and deepen knowledge

- **Decide quickly:** organizing cross-functional team workshops to collaborate and share knowledge, drive integration and delivery of solutions

- **Orient toward a journey of change:** valuing change as a path toward equilibrium, not as a destination

- **Align strategies and manage talent:** optimizing talents and expertise (Baran & Woznyj, 2019).

Practice: Mindful Agility

"Being a relational leader who is mindful of inclusion requires being agile in alignment and coordination of meaning and action with others" (Gallegos, 2013, p. 187). Gallegos senses the tension between the status quo and inclusive leadership. Explore why agility might be required when confronting opposing principles or core beliefs. Reflect upon a time when you had to negotiate a decision from two or multiple parties who held opposing principles. How might humble inquiry and deep listening reveal a common ground? How might mindfulness and agility practices offer clarity and directions for the collective leadership?

Inclusive Leadership

The importance of community resilience and inclusive leadership is not a new idea. For more than a decade, community development scholars have noted that community resilience resides with the balance of community capital and an emphasis on the people with the social capital (Callaghan & Colton, 2008). Enhancing the capacity of communities to manage adversities, social unrest, and disasters involves drawing upon the interconnections, shared resources, social interactions, problem solving (Robinson & Carson, 2016; Shenk, Krejci, Passe, 2019), interests, and expertise of all community members. How to include and engage the diverse membership of communities, though, has had less attention.

Inclusive leaders model humility and courage (Gallegos, 2013). They share power throughout the community. In turn, residents report feeling valued and respected for their perspective. From inclusivity, a collective identity is fostered; a "co-created compelling vision aligns work with higher purpose and greater good" (Geller, 2009, p. 189). They speak out against incidents of "structural inequity, and making change to long-standing traditions and organizational practices needs to be a part of a leader's toolkit if real and sustainable change is to be fostered" (Gallegos, 2013, p. 179). They pay attention to the implicit power and privilege within hierarchies and ask for inquiry and listening from those in higher positions. They set boundaries for expected behavior during individual and system interactions.

These attributes open the heart for empathy and collaboration. The inclusive leader enacts the inclusion of all residents at the individual, relational, and system levels. Multiple perspectives and areas of expertise are essential during uncertainty. This inclusion shifts the nature of attention by learning to hear differently. Leaders bend their hearing to learn something they don't know. They show empathy while listening. They attempt to embody diverse perspectives as to generate future possibilities. Hearing diverse perspectives also requires observing the interplay of people and practices. Leaders look for patterns that emerge among players and throughout the system. Inclusive leadership involves paying attention to who is talking, whose perspective is needed, and the limitations to really seeing an issue. They must be willing to disrupt preferences based upon familiarity and history. Through the inclusion and listening, leaders become altered by the experience.

Resilient communities are dependent upon their leaders' capacity for leading into the future. Leading into the future requires letting go of self-concepts that may be products of former ways of thinking and becoming. Leading in turbulence requires leaders to shift their position from being at the center of power and decision making to sharing them with residents. Leaders are open to revising their identities and mindsets. Leaders of resilient communities forge into complexity with mindfulness, agility, and inclusivity. They favor suspending prejudgments with an observing mind and generating cocreated dialogue through humble inquiry and deep listening. They value positive, authentic communication as a way to foster trusting relationships. Through relationships, leaders open their hearts to inclusive relationships and open their will to dismantle structures of inequities. For with these collective, dialogic relationships comes the community's resilience in times of complexity and uncertainty.

Case Study
Community Resilience in Times of Turbulence

In the evening news, the community learns that a young Black man has died at the scene of an alleged crime. Videotapes reveal that the man, accompanied by his girlfriend, was shopping in the local Dollar General store. While shopping the two appear to have a disagreement and from that point it appears that the two begin shouting at one another. At this time, the video shows that the store manager approaches the two and talks with them. The man becomes agitated and pushes the store manager. The manager walks quickly away, and the man and woman resume their interaction. A few minutes later, a police officer approaches the couple. He talks with them. The man appears to become more agitated by throwing his hands in the air and by grabbing cans off of the shelf. The young man picks up a can and throws it down the aisle. The can hits a bystander.

The police officer then puts his hand on his gun still in the holster, stretches out his arm, and holds up his hand. It appears he tells the man to stop. The man at this time turns and runs down the aisle away from the police officer, who then takes chase. The camera angle changes at this time, and the film then shows the two running down a back aisle. A customer and his basket get in the way of the fleeing man who then stumbles and falls. The police officer is quickly upon the man and attempts to handcuff him. They scuffle. The film then shows the young Black man overpowering the police office, putting him in a chokehold and pulling a knife. From behind the scuffling two men, a woman officer is immediately upon the two and kicks the knife from the man and pushes him off of the police office. The officers then team up on the Black man and restrain him by holding him to the floor. He resists again, so the male officer puts his knee in the neck of the young man, pinning him to the floor. The young man makes some movements and then lies still. The film later shows paramedics arriving, attempting to revive the man and then leaving with him on a stretcher. The Police Department later reports the young Black man died at the scene. The film will not be released until an investigation has been completed.

Within the week, Black Lives Matter assemblies begin, and a statement is released by the Ministry Alliance:

> Justice and equity are the pillars of community development. No one in our community is disposable; our voices and lives have value. Today, we remember the families of George Floyd, Breonna Taylor, and, our brother, Amari Davis. We mourn the lives of people who have been extrajudicially murdered by the state. We are frustrated and disappointed in our community and everyone who has again

> watched those charged to protect us casually take the lives of our neighbors. Black lives matter, and Black people must be protected from police brutality. Our communities deserve better and we will not rest until our vision for a community committed to justice, equity, and our collective well-being is realized.
>
> The president of the local university sends out a public letter chastising the action of the community police department and supports their Office of Diversity. University students join local assemblies. Traffic is blocked by demonstrators, and business owners demand something be done with those they call "troublemakers." The investigation concludes, and all police officers are cleared of any wrongdoing.
>
> How might you assist your community in this turbulent situation? What type of leadership approach would you take? What values would you want to uphold while engaged in leading? How might mindfulness, agility, and inclusivity guide your leadership approach? What would your plan be? With whom? How would you execute the plan?

References

Alvesson, M. & Willmott, H. (2002). Identity regulation as organizational control: Producing the appropriate individual. *Journal of Management Studies, 39,* 619–644.

Baran, B.E. & Woznyj, H.M. (2019). Managing VUCA: The human dynamics of agility. *Organizational Dynamic,* https://doi.org/10.1016/j.orgdyn.2020.100787

Birkinshaw, J. (2018). What to expect from agile. *MIT Sloan Management Review,* 8–11.

Bolden, R. (2011). Distributed leadership in organizations: A review of theory and research. *International Journal of Management Reviews, 13*(3). https://doi.org/10.1111/j.1468-2370.2011.00306.x

Bono, J.E., Schen, W. & Snyder, M. (2010). Fostering integrative community leadership. *The Leadership Quarterly, 21* (2), 324–335.

Brown, V.A., Harris, J.A. & Russell, J.Y. (2010). *Tackling wicked problems through the transdisciplinary imagination.* Earthscan from Routledge.

Callaghan, E.G. & Colton, J. (2008). Building sustainable and resilient communities: A balancing act of community capital. *Environment, Development and Sustainability*, 10(6), 931–942.

Centers for Disease Control and Prevention (CDC). (2020). *Overweight & obesity*. https://www.cdc.gov/obesity/data/prevalence-maps.html

Crosby, B.C. & Bryson, J. (2005). *Leadership for the common good: Tackling public problems in a shared-power world*. John Wiley & Sons.

Cullen-Lester, K.L. & Yammarino, F.J. (2016). Collective and network approaches to leadership: Special issue introduction. *The Leadership Quarterly 27*(2), 173–180.

Cyert, R.M. (1990). Defining leadership and explicating the process. *Nonprofit Management and Leadership, 1*(1). https://doi.org/10.1002/nml.4130010105

Endres, S. & Weibler, J. (2017). Towards a three-component model of relational social constructionist leadership: A systematic review and critical interpretive synthesis. *International Journal of Management Reviews, 19*, 214–236.

Gallegos, P.V. (2013). The work of inclusive leadership: Fostering authentic relationships, modeling courage and humility. In B.M. Ferdman. (Ed.), *Diversity at work: The practice of inclusion*. John Wiley & Sons.

Geller, K. (2009). Transformative learning dynamics for developing relational leaders. In B. Fisher-Yoshida, D.D. Geller & S.A. Schapiro (Eds.), *Innovations in transformative learning: Space, culture, and the arts* (pp. 177–201). Peter Lang.

Heiftez, R.A. & Laurie, D.L. (2001). The work of leadership. *Harvard Business Review*, 124–134.

Ibarra, H. (1999). Provisional selves: Experimenting with image and identity in professional adaptation. *Administrative Science Quarterly, 44*, 764–791.

Ivory, G. (2015). Developing a leadership platform. In G. Ivory, A. Hyle, R. McClellan & M. Acker-Hocevar. (Eds.). *Quandaries of the small-district superintendency*. Palgrave Macmillan. https://link.springer.com/chapter/10.1057/9781137363251_2.

Johansen, B. (2017). *The new leadership literacies: Thriving in a future of extreme disruption and distributed everything*. Berrett-Koehler.

Judge, T.A., Bono, J.E., Ilies, R., Gerhardt, M.W. (2002). Personality and leadership: A qualitative and quantitative review. *Journal of Applied Psychology, 87*(4), 765–780.

Kouzes, J.M. & Posner, B.Z. (2017). *The leadership challenge: How to make extraordinary things happen in organizations*. John Wiley & Sons.

Offermann, L.R. & Coats, M.R. (2018). Implicit theories of leadership: Stability and change over two decades. *The Leadership Quarterly, 29*(4), 513–522.

Plowman, D. & Duchon, D. (2008). Dispelling the myths about leadership: From cybernetics to emergence. In M. Uhl-Bein & M. Ross (Eds.), *Complexity leadership, Part I: Conceptual Foundations (pp. 129-153)*. Information Age Publishing.

Robinson, G.M. & Carson, D.A. (2016). Resilient communities: Transitions, pathways and resourcefulness. *The Geographic Journal*, 1–9.

Scharmer, C.O. (2018). *The essentials of theory U: Core principles and applications*. Berrett-Koehler.

Scharmer, C.O. (2016). *Theory U: Leading from the future as it emerges*. Berrett-Koehler.

Schein, E.H. (2013). *Humble inquiry: The gentle art of asking instead of telling*. Berrett-Koehler.

Schweigert, F.J. (2007). Learning to lead: Strengthening the practice of community leadership. *Leadership, 3*(3), 325–342.

Senge, P., Scharmer, C.O., Jaworski, J. & Flowers, B.S. (2014). *Presence: Human purpose and the field of the future*. Crown Business.

Shamir, B. & Eilam, G. (2005). 'What's your story?' A life-stories approach to authentic leadership development. *The Leadership Quarterly, 16*(3), 395–417.

Shenk, L., Krejci, C. & Passe, U. (2019). Agents of change—together: Using agent-based models to inspire social capital building for resilient communities. *Community Development, 50*(2), 256–272.

Silsbee, D. (2018). *Presence-based leadership: Complexity for clarity, resilience, and results that matter*. Yes! Global Inc.

Stone, A.G. and Patterson, K. (2005) "The history of leadership focus": Servant leadership roundtable. Virginia Beach, VA: Regent University.

Taylor, B. (2010). Do you pass the leadership test? *Leadership*. https://hbr.org/2010/08/pass-leadership-test

Uhl-Bien, M. & Marion, R. (2009). Meso modeling of leadership: Integrating micro- and macro-perspectives of leadership. *The Leadership Quarterly*, doi: 10.1016/j.leaqua.2009.04.007

Marketing Your Community

Amanda Sutt & Valerie Kinney

Community marketing is essential to successful economic development. Learn economic development marketing principles and how to recruit new firms to your community. Become familiar with the elements of a marketing plan, including goals, objectives and strategic action steps, budget and resource requirements, and the roles and responsibilities of participating organizations and stakeholders.

Learning Outcomes

- Participants will learn the three audiences for community marketing: internal audience, partners, and external audience.

- Participants will review community branding and reputation, marketing "musts," and effective marketing tools and avenues.

- Participants will study building community buy-in in the marketing process.

You can't just expect people to happen upon your community and immediately fall in love, drop everything, and move there. It would be nice if they did, but you have to give them something more persuasive to compel them to action. What are they missing out on if they don't invest their businesses and lives into your community? That's where a solid community marketing plan comes into play. Marketing your community is not that dissimilar to marketing a business or a product. The 7Ps of marketing (*product, place, promotion, price, process, people,* and *physical evidence*) still apply with some adjustments to how we view product and price.

1. **Product:** The product is your community or the service that your organization offers to support your community.

2. **Place:** The place is the sum of the marketing channels you use to promote your community, your service, and your ideas.

3. **Promotion:** Promotion is the sum of the tactics you implement to share your message (e.g., advertising, events, social media, email).

4. **Price:** This is more complicated when it comes to community development if you are not exchanging a service for a fee. If you don't have a service for a fee, the price then falls to items such as taxes, incentives, property value, and cost of living that a business locating and operating in your community must incur.

5. **Process:** The process is made up of the steps a business would experience to relocate to or start up in your community.

6. **People:** The people are the personal interactions businesses have as they interact with your community as they decide whether to do business in your community.

7. **Physical Evidence:** Physical evidence is key with service-based marketing and includes items such as your website, brochures, and signage to highlight your offerings and tell your story.

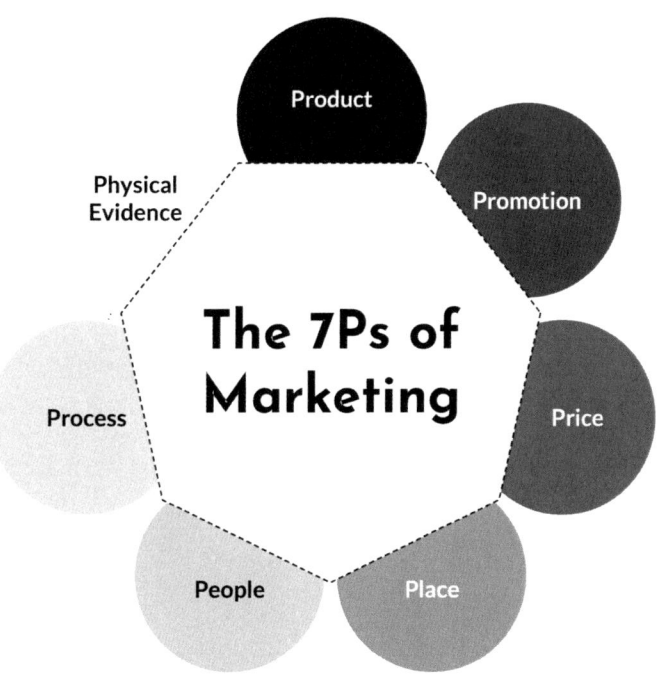

Looking at each marketing principle individually is important to understand marketing, but this abstracted view can be hard to hold together as you start to apply this to your community.

To help explain what marketing looks like today and how these principles work together to promote your community, we borrow concepts introduced by Allan Dibb (2018) to illustrate what goes into a very popular community event—a farmer's market.

- If you make a sign promoting the event, that is advertising.

- If you have a person dressed up as a carrot dancing on a busy street flipping a sign for the farmer's market, that is promotion.

- If the dancing carrot fills in as the school crossing-guard and people start tweeting about it, that is public relations.

- If the local newspaper writes an article based on the trending tweets, that is publicity.

- If people come to the farmer's market, talk to the vendors about their offerings, and buy, that is sales.

- And if you planned the entire thing, that is marketing.

With a clearer view of what marketing looks like, you need to know what it takes to get there. There are three critical elements that you need in place before you hire your dancing carrot—your brand, your audience, and your plan.

Branding Your Community

Now that you have a picture of what marketing is, and before you market to recruit new firms, you need to know who you are as a community. You need to establish your brand and understand how this is separate from marketing. Your brand encompasses your vision and reputation, while marketing consists of your tactics and the progress your efforts produce.

Branding is the manifestation of your beliefs and is displayed through your community, experiences, and interactions with your residents as well as the outside world. It is how your audience connects with your community and ultimately how it makes them feel. Your brand can be found not only in these touch points, but also in a logo, website, written materials, and more.

Five Steps to Establish Your Brand

Your brand should reflect who you are and what you want to be and connect with the audiences that you want to attract and retain. The graphic below illustrates a five-step process for building an intentional brand for your community. Even if you have not engaged in a formal branding process, you *have* a brand, so these steps can help you add intentionality to your brand.

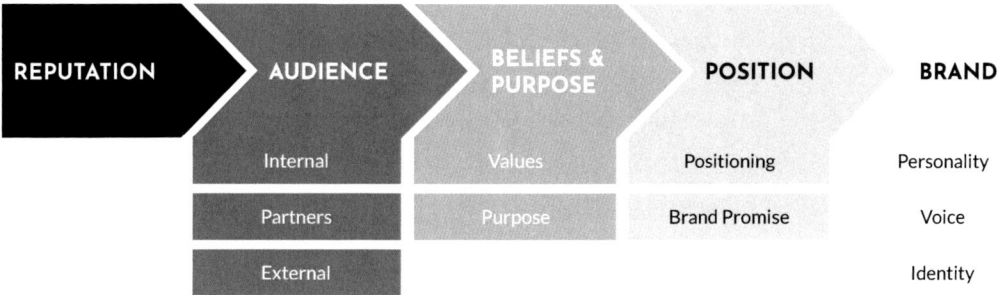

1. **Uncover your reputation:** Before you dive into clarifying what you want your brand to become, it is essential to understand how people currently perceive your community to determine your current reputation. You can easily collect this information through surveys, interviews, and focus groups.

    This is a critical first step to get buy-in from your current community and to create alignment as you begin to market. This is especially true if your reputation does not reflect your reality. You will need to address this gap to clarify where the disconnect is stemming from. By addressing and mending this gap, it will give you a more solid foundation for clarifying or repositioning your brand. At the end of the day, it does not matter how much you like your brand; it only matters what other people think of it.

2. **Define your audiences:** Community development is about helping people, so you need to understand who you are serving. When you are talking about branding and marketing a community and start to consider your audience, it is very easy to confuse who you are serving, the roles people take, and resources these unique groups can bring to the table. When you talk about a community, you are talking about a lot of different people. It helps to break them into three categories: internal audience, partners, and external audience.

    - **Internal audience:** Anyone within your office or organization, as well as community members, which can include elected officials, chambers of commerce, state leaders, and nonprofits, is your internal audience. It is critical to get alignment with your internal audience so that you have a consistent message about your community, no matter whom prospective businesses may talk to. It takes a lot less effort—and you can make a lot more progress—when everyone moves in the same direction.

    - **Partners:** This is any person or organization that will put in a similar effort and receive similar benefit to your marketing work. Depending on your internal audience, your partners can include any agency that supports you and will mutually benefit from your actions. This can also include elected officials, chambers, and nonprofits if you are coordinating with them as a collective to attract and retain business and support the community.

- **External audience:** This is anyone that you want to attract to your community. This could include new residents as well as new businesses or organizations that will boost the local economy and bring new jobs and growth.

Target Audience #1:

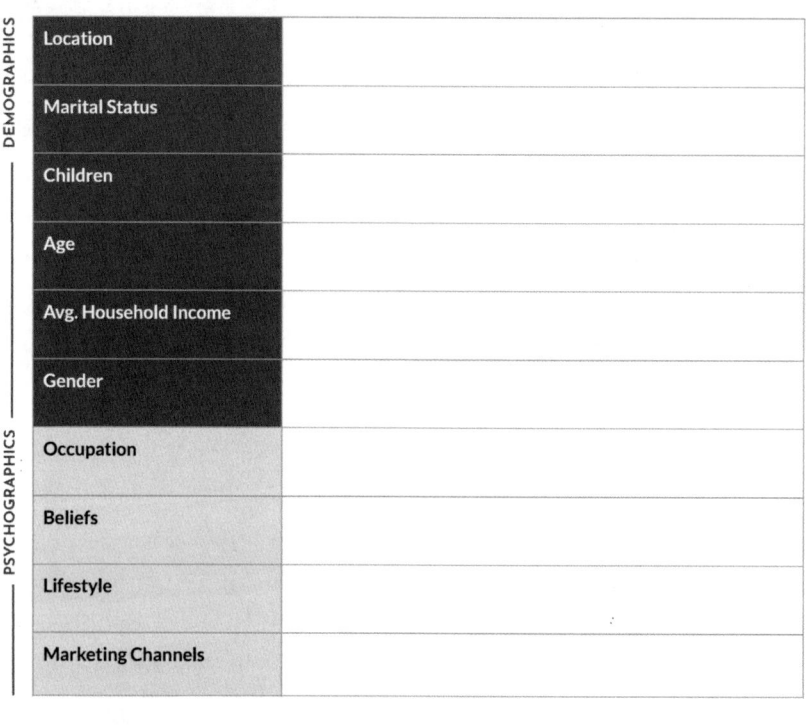

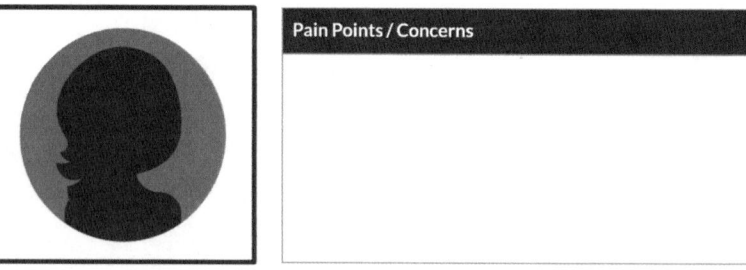

You will want to create a profile for each audience you have identified. An audience profile is a quick summary of the demographics and psychographics of these people in an easy-to-share format. It may help to think of audience profiles as stereotypical representations of the types of people included in an audience that help you better understand who these people are, where they are coming from, and how they think. You need these profiles in your toolbox to help you better connect with your audience members and maximize your resources to reach them where they are, rather than aiming a message in a general direction and running the risk of your audience missing it. As you start to define each audience, know that you may have multiple profiles per audience segment. If the needs in an audience are very different and you need to communicate with them in a unique approach, it would be worth breaking out a subgroup.

Demographic information can be pulled from data sources such as local government data or the U.S. Census Bureau, American FactFinder, and the Urban Institute. The psychographics, which include the attitudes, aspirations, and other psychological criteria, on the other hand are a little more difficult to collect. If resources are available, you can hire a market research firm to collect this data or you can start with your own observations. If you do the latter, for each audience you will need to answer: What would they want or look for in a community? What are their values? What do you need from them? The goal is to not only think about your audience in terms of their demographics but also their world view and how they navigate the world each day so you can better understand and speak to their needs and how your product can make a difference in their lives (Jiwa, 2014).

If you start with your observations, you will need to make sure that you build systems to collect this information moving forward. Collecting feedback gives you an even greater insight into your audience's world and the challenges they are currently facing, allowing you to speak to their pain points and share how what you have to offer can make their lives better. When the average American is coming in contact with 6,000 to 10,000 ads per day (Carr, 2020), knowing and speaking to your audience's pain will help your message stand out. The good news is that collecting feedback from your audience can be relatively inexpensive, thanks to free and inexpensive resources available for conducting polls and surveys; you can also collect feedback through phone calls, feedback boxes on your website, or even using the live video feature on social media.

3. **Clarify your beliefs and purpose:** It is very easy to copy the look and feel of any other community or organization, but it will not have the same success if beliefs and passion are not present to support the visuals. Your beliefs and purpose are the foundation that your brand and marketing will build on. This is who you already are as a community, but so often this is assumed and not documented. It is a part of your oral culture, but when you write this down and

start to clarify what you want, other people can more easily share this as well. This step of branding may have already been established in other steps of your community's vision so do not feel like you have to recreate the wheel if you already have this in place.

- **Values:** Your values encompass what is important in life to your community and are shaped in communities by your history and culture. With the rate at which the world is changing, it can be very easy to get swept up in a new trend and lose track of what makes you special and unique. Having values helps you stay the course as well as attract residents and businesses who share these same values. Knowing your values will make positioning and building your brand much easier.

- **Purpose:** Your purpose is the reason you exist and drives your vision for where you are going as a community. To borrow a phrase popularized by Jim Collins and Jerry Portas (1994), this can be a BHAG—big, hairy, audacious goal—but it needs to be grounded in the audience and values you already have in place. As you get into your marketing plan, you will start to break your purpose and vision into smaller milestones with your goals and objectives to turn these ideas into a reality.

4. **Your position:** Once you know whom you are serving, what you believe, and where you are going, you then need to refine the path that you want to take in order to grow. Although your choices are infinite as you move forward, your goal is to continue to build on the work that you have started so that you have a community and brand that people remember and want to join.

    - **Positioning:** The goal with positioning a community is to leverage and promote your strengths that align with your vision in a unique way to attract the people and businesses you want. You may want to do a competitive analysis at this point to see what you are up against, but don't get so wrapped up in this that you position your community in a potential gap in the market and lose track of who you are at your core.

    - **Brand promise:** Your brand promise is the experience or value you want people to have with your community each and every time. This should be simple and easy to share and remember. This consistent experience is what builds trust and your reputation.

5. **Build your brand:** Building a brand *after* you have completed Steps 1 through 4 makes building the public-facing elements much easier. You have built the

depth and purpose that supports the visual elements as well as started the buy-in process so that your community will get behind your brand and work together.

- **Brand personality:** Just as an individual has a personality that distinguishes them, your brand has a personality that distinguishes you from other communities. You can use the exact same adjectives to describe your community as you would a person. Be sure to include a short description that clarifies the personality. For example, different generations have different pictures for *professional*; a Baby Boomer may envision a person in a suit at a desk, whereas a Millennial may define *professional* as the caliber of work and not the way they look.

- **Brand voice:** Your brand voice is the way your brand sounds and should include four traits: *character, tone, language,* and *purpose*. The character of your voice can pull from your brand personality. The tone focuses on the feeling that you want your language to portray. The language describes the style of words you use, for example, complex or simple. Finally, the purpose defines the goal of your content (such as educating, entertaining, or informing).

- **Brand identity:** So often, communities want to start branding by designing a new logo, but this is actually the last step. Shapes, colors, textures, and styles come very easily when you know who you are as a brand. Your brand identity can include your logo, colors, fonts, tagline, stationery, imagery, icons, textures, and brand standards, to name a few.

Marketing Your Community

Marketing is how you get your message and story into the world in a way that connects. It starts with keeping your audience top of mind and creating content that provides them with real value. Marketing is much easier when your brand has been clearly established; now you know your audience look, feel, and tone in a way that enables you to focus on getting your message out and connecting with your audience to achieve your goals. If you have done the branding work, then you know, without a doubt, that your community will embrace the dancing carrot idea for your farmer's market. But before you dive into marketing and start placing ads and posting messages on social media, you need to have a plan. Similar to branding your community, the creative piece of the logo comes last, and the creative for your marketing follows suit.

For your marketing to achieve the results you want, you need to have a plan. You wouldn't start building a house without blueprints, so why try to market without a plan? When you have a clear vision of what you are building or creating, you can share that with your team to think through what you really need. Together, you can also think about what you want and can even consider given challenges that exist, so you are prepared to tackle them as they come. This may also help you understand where you need buy-in. Your marketing plan is essentially your playbook for getting your message out into the world and in front of your intended audience to achieve your goals. Having a clear marketing plan empowers your internal audience and partners to understand what you are doing, where you want to go, and when they can take action to support your goals.

Planning ahead also allows you to be proactive and anticipate needs rather than reacting as situations arise, which can really stall your progress. When it comes to marketing, if you plan ahead, you can share the reality of your situation and give your audience a very transparent, genuine answer rather than feeling the need to defend yourself and your actions because you had to come up with a solution at the last second.

Your marketing plan should cover a set duration. The typical duration is six months to three years, with most averaging twelve months to match your fiscal year.

Your marketing plan should include the following elements:

- Audiences
- Goals
- Objectives
- Strategies
- Tactics
- Resources & Budget
- Schedule

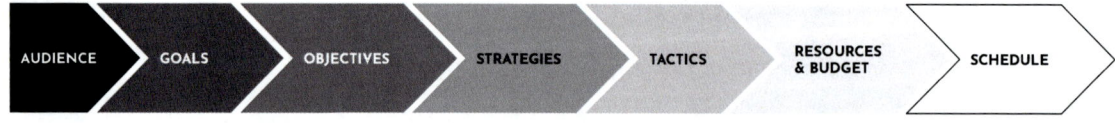

Audiences

You can pull your audience profiles from your branding work. Be sure to consider all audiences, because some of your efforts may include marketing to your internal audience or partners before you market to your external audience to get their buy-in.

PRO TIP: Each time you create a new marketing plan is also a great opportunity to review your audience profiles to make any necessary revisions.

Goals

Goals are the results that you want to achieve. Goal setting is an important first step in crafting your marketing plan because it helps you not only clarify what you want your efforts to achieve but will also help you focus your efforts to help you see your success.

Take the duration of the marketing plan into account and determine what you would like your community to look like at the end of this period. You can leverage your long-term vision and match those milestones with your marketing plan, if applicable. If your vision does not lend itself to your milestones, you can start with a SWOT analysis to examine your community's *Strengths, Weaknesses, Opportunities, and Threats*. This can ensure that your marketing goals support the change you want to make happen. A SWOT analysis will help ground your goals in your current reality so that you are setting yourself up for success.

When creating your goals, you need to make sure they are specific and clear for everyone involved to take action and make progress. Chances are you may have heard of SMART (Specific, Measurable, Action-oriented, Realistic, Time-bound) goals before; Michael Hyatt has improved the goal-setting process with his SMARTER goals, which take motivation and buy-in from your team into account as well (Hyatt, 2018). Goals that are considered SMARTER are:

- **Specific** to focus and direct your energies on a tangible result;
- **Measurable** so you can keep track of your progress to know if your efforts are working or not;
- **Actionable** with a clear initiating verb that prompts specific activity;
- **Risky** enough to leverage your natural tendency to rise to challenges;
- **Time-keyed** so you are prompted exactly when to act;
- **Exciting** to inspire and harness the power of your intrinsic motivation, this should be something you WANT to do;
- **Relevant** within the overall context of your community's stage of life (such as newly organized, branded, or recovering from a crisis).

Once you have your goals in place and have checked them against the SMARTER system, you're ready to start thinking about the path you'll use to reach them, which starts with your objectives and strategy.

PRO TIP: Don't go overboard! Start with two to four goals that you would like to see in the next six to twelve months. Keep this process simple so you are setting yourself up for success instead of failure.

Objectives

Objectives are used to measure progress as you work toward your goal. This includes determining what success looks like for your community. Success can sometimes be subjective, so it's important to define this up front so everyone is on the same page and has the same expectations. When you know what success looks like, you need to determine how you'll measure it.

Part of measuring success includes mapping out where you want to be by the end of the set period you are working in (i.e. the next six months, one year, etc.), defining the return on investment you are looking for, and setting milestones for checking in on your progress.

It is critical to understand the role the objectives play in your marketing plan. The world is changing faster than at any other point in history, so you need to be able to test new ideas and strategies, as well as know when past methods are no longer relevant. Objectives let you know when your plans and theories are working or not; if they are not working, then you can change your process. It's important to note that failure is a critical element of success; you can learn just as much through what went wrong, but you need to see the value in the lesson learned so that you change your course to stay focused on your goal.

PRO TIP: As with your goals, don't overcomplicate this so that you are spending more time measuring than implementing. Work with your team to determine key performance indicators that will tell you if your efforts are working or not. Over time, you may determine that you need to add or remove indicators if they are not helping you understand if the effort you are making is supporting the change you want to make.

Strategies

Your strategy is the approach you take to achieve your goal. *Merriam-Webster* defines strategy as "a careful plan or method" and "the art of devising or employing plans or stratagems toward a goal" ("Strategy," n.d.). Creating your strategy is a natural next step after setting your goals and objectives because this will help you start to establish how you want to get to your desired end result. Don't confuse strategy with tactics, though. Tactics are the specific actions you'll take to follow your strategy in order to meet your goals.

As with goals, an established strategy is a key part of your marketing plan because it helps your leadership team and anyone else involved in your efforts work from the same starting point. It enables you to allocate your resources and efforts as well as begin defining roles so each team member knows what he or she is responsible for contributing. With no strategy in place, you lack the basic guidance necessary for making sure your team understands the goals at hand and how you hope to achieve them.

Marketing and selling your community is just as much, if not more, about your approach and building relationships with your audience than it is about the number of leads in your pipeline and conversion rates. Relationships allow you to build trust with your audience, and if you don't have their trust, conversion becomes much more difficult if not impossible. One of the easiest ways to build trust with an audience is through the consistent information you share with them.

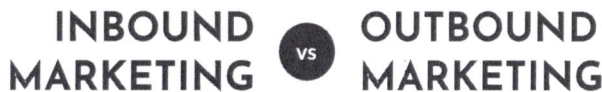

PRO TIP: When you are considering the best approaches to attract new firms to your community, you will want to take into consideration the way your decision makers prefer to get their information as well as when you should choose to use outbound vs. inbound marketing. *Outbound marketing* is your more traditional method of broadcasting what you have to offer. *Inbound marketing* is the process of attracting, delighting, and engaging your customers.

Tactics

Your tactics are the action steps, or marketing tools, you'll use to achieve your goals and objectives. Tactics can cover everything from email marketing to social media content, a PR plan, video, advertising, and more—essentially any point at which your brand and message can connect with your audience. Each strategy that you define should include the tactics that you plan to implement.

The marketing industry has exploded in the last few decades with the amount of tools you have available, and it continues to grow. The following is a broad summary of the tactics that you may want to consider in your plan.

- **Digital advertising:** The use of online and other digital channels such as social media, apps, and search engines to share promotional content with an audience is considered digital advertising.

  - **Social media advertising:** Social media advertising is a form of digital advertising in which a business or organization places ads on social networking sites, typically for the purpose of either raising brand awareness or generating a response from those who view their ads. Social media can either be categorized as organic content, meaning there is no cost to the advertiser to post optimized content for the audience to interact with, or it can be categorized as paid advertising. Paid social media ads allow advertisers to pay a fee to target their content to specific audiences (such as specific age groups or people in certain zip codes) that they are not able to reach with organic content.

  - **Display advertising:** Display advertising uses graphic or text banner ads that are displayed in very specific locations on a website or social media platform, typically used to raise awareness about a product or service.

  - **Geofencing:** This method of digital advertising uses location-based services such as GPS, cellular data, and Wi-Fi to define a specific geographic boundary within which to trigger an ad to be displayed when someone enters the virtual boundary.

  - **Pay-per-click:** Pay-per-click, or PPC, is a form of advertising in which advertisers pay when a viewer clicks on one of their ads.

  - **Online directories:** Similar to the Yellow Pages, online directories provide the opportunity to advertise your business or organization in specific internet-based directories.

  - **SEO:** Search engine optimization (SEO) is a method for improving a website's ranking on search engines to improve the likelihood of a new user finding the site. It employs high-quality, keyword-rich content, decreased page load times, optimized images, and other features that make the site attractive to search engines.

  - **Direct response:** Direct response is a form of marketing in which advertisers use calls to action to generate a more immediate response from the audience.

- **Customer relation scripts and team training:** Using customer relation scripts provides team members with a consistent message so that no matter who an audience member speaks with, they hear the same message. These scripts are very useful when training new hires or brand ambassadors so they can immediately onboard and become more familiar with the brand and how it needs to be portrayed.

- **Direct mail** (such as postcards, newsletters, or brochures)**:** Direct mail marketing uses items that are printed and traditionally mailed to a specific audience.

- **Events:** Events can include any activity where the community is welcome to gather and interact, such as fairs, holiday festivities, farmers' markets, parades, sporting events, and fundraisers. As a result of the COVID-19 pandemic in 2020, many shifted to virtual gatherings or events that adhere to social distancing guidelines in order to prevent the spread of illness. Events provide the opportunity for community members to experience the brand firsthand.

  - **Event sponsorship:** Communities often sponsor events through monetary donations, time, services, or branded items that help raise awareness and grow the organization's network.

  - **Trade shows:** Trade shows are industry-specific events where timely information can be shared on relevant topics, innovations, new products, and more. Most trade shows include a vendor expo where sponsors and other industry-related vendors may interact with attendees to share information about their products, service, and solutions.

  - **Open houses:** An open house is an event hosted by a business or organization where members of the public are invited inside to learn more about the entity's mission and offerings.

  - **Webinars, seminars, and presentations:** Seminars and presentations offer the opportunity to educate an audience on any given subject and usually include a time for questions and answers. Webinars are the virtual version of a seminar, typically taking place in real time and allowing viewers to join the event from any location.

  - **Networking:** Engaging with a group of people for professional or social purposes to exchange contact information and share experience is one of the oldest and most effective means of marketing.

- **Inbound marketing:** Inbound marketing is the act of extending focused content to a qualified list of prospects where they are with valuable messages they didn't know they needed.

  - **Ads:** Ads—or the practice of advertising—utilize placements in print and digital media to promote a brand, business, product, or service in order to build interest and generate leads.

  - **Automated email marketing:** The process of sending emails to customers or prospects, usually triggered by a specific action, can include several types of messages, including transactional emails (such as a *Welcome* or *Thank You* email) as well as reminder emails (e.g., "Don't forget about this weekend's farmers market!") and other drip emails that share a series of content on specific topics. Oftentimes, automated emails are used in inbound marketing to nurture leads with additional information that addresses your audience's pain points.

  - **SEO and blogs:** *See above definition for SEO under Digital advertising.* In inbound marketing, SEO is used to generate leads to be nurtured. Blogs are online publications, written about specific topics by one or more authors, that are optimized for searchability based on specific keywords potential leads may be researching online.

  - **Social media:** Social media encompasses websites and mobile applications that allow users to create and share content with family and friends, as well as follow influencers, brands, and causes that matter to them. Content posted to social media can be used to better inform and support leads as they go through the decision-making process.

  - **Surveys:** Surveys are a method of research for collecting information from current leads and audience members about specific topics, their experience with a specific event, product, or service, and other information. Often, surveys are used to improve the support and content a business or organization is delivering.

  - **Videos:** Videos can be used to educate, entertain, and inform an audience on any topic related to your brand, products, services, and more. Adding videos on your website can aid in increasing your site's ranking on search engines and help you attract quality leads. Like social media content, videos can be used as a way to provide information to leads and support them in their decision-making process.

- **Public relations:** The Public Relations Society of America (PRSA) defines public relations as "a strategic communication process that builds mutually beneficial relationships between organizations and their publics" (Public Relations Society of America, n.d.).

    - **Press release:** a written communication sent to targeted media outlets that reports specific but brief information about an event or other newsworthy topic

    - **Feature article:** an in-depth look at a topic, product, or industry generally featured around human interest

    - **Product announcement:** content created specifically for promoting a new product and distributed through a variety of channels

    - **Email marketing:** the creation and distribution of consistent updates to a list of subscribers about new information and current events so the company can stay top of mind and provide opportunities for engagement and interaction

    - **Newsletter:** an informal publication (printed or digital) circulated to subscribers on a regular basis (i.e. monthly, quarterly, etc.)

    - **Speech:** an opportunity to give an oral presentation in front of a captive audience who could benefit from your knowledge and expertise

    - **Annual report:** a comprehensive report on an organization's activities throughout the past year, typically to provide stakeholders with information about the organization's activities and financial performance

    - **Community sponsorship:** support of a local event through monetary donations, time, services, or branded items

    - **Charitable donations:** providing support to nonprofit organizations through monetary donations, goods, time, or services to help the organization reach its goals

- **Print advertising:** Print advertising involves placing ads in a variety of publications and other printed media. Print advertising can include imagery and graphics as well as messaging that includes a call to action to encourage the audience to take the desired next steps.

- **Promotional materials:** can include printed items such as fliers, posters, coupons, and business cards as well as pens, koozies, notepads, and other merchandise that includes a business or organization's logo

- **Table tents:** a self-standing promotional item typically placed on a table, desk, counter, or other flat surface and often used in restaurants, trade show booths, hotels, and other places where marketing communication might be beneficial

- **Brochures:** printed pieces that are evergreen and can serve as a lasting reference that provides informational content that helps your audience take action

- **Flier:** a single-sheet print piece that promotes an organization and/or its products or services

- **Billboards:** Large format outdoor signage for advertising generally found along busy roadways

- **Publications:** printed works such as newspapers and magazines that often include a mix of articles, editorials, and advertisements. Publications to consider include:

  - **Industry publications:** Often referred to as a trade journal or trade magazine, this type of publication is targeted to audience members in a specific trade or industry, providing them with timely updates and developments.

  - **National publications:** National publications can include newspapers and magazines, as well as trade publications, with no specific geographic target for distribution and can be printed daily, weekly, monthly, quarterly, annually or at other intervals.

  - **Regional publications:** Regional publications can include newspapers, magazines, and other works that include news and other information specific to a defined area such as a group of counties. Such publications may be printed weekly, monthly, quarterly, biannually, annually, or at other frequencies.

  - **Local newspapers:** These publications include reports on local events and news, as well as editorials, feature articles, and advertisements that are generally specific to a certain geographic area. Local newspapers are often published either daily or weekly.

- **Trade directories:** Trade directories are a type of business listing specific to a particular industry or trade that include a business's name as well as its address, phone number, offerings, total employees, and years in operation. Some online trade directories also include opportunities for comments and reviews for each business.

- **Signage:** The use of visual graphics to share a message with the public.

  - **Banners:** This type of signage can be used indoors or outdoors for many purposes. Banners can be made out of a variety of materials and often include metal grommets in each corner for hanging displays.

  - **Murals and wraps:** These eye-catching tools can be used to enhance offices, stores, communities, and more with product information and/or marketing messages, and can also provide life-sized representations of what you have to offer.

  - **Window graphics and decals:** These signs used for advertising or marketing purposes are placed directly on a window that can be usually customized in color, shape, size, and style to promote available locations or plans for development.

  - **Monument signs:** This type of free-standing sign is usually placed low to the ground and made of weather-resistant materials that often serve as wayfinders to direct people to a specific business or organization's physical location or to mark a geographic area.

  - **Yard signs:** Often called lawn signs, yard signs are made of durable materials and can be used for a variety of purposes in outdoor settings for business promotion, real estate, general information, and more.

  - **Digital or electronic signs:** This signage employs the use of LEDs, LCDs, and other illumination techniques to display information, imagery, media, video, and other content and often provide directions, advertising and marketing messages, and more.

- **Social media:** Social media content is used to help keep a profile active and the audience engaged with a business or brand, as well as raise awareness about particular products, services, or information. The content should educate or entertain first, and then sell. Please note that these platforms are subject to change due to the rapid nature of the content and shifts to meet user demand, so check recent resources for the most up-to-date details on these platforms—and others yet to be developed.

- **Facebook:** This is one of the world's most popular social networking sites that enables users to connect with friends and family by sharing status updates, images, videos, and other newsworthy items of interest.

- **YouTube:** YouTube is a social video-sharing platform and the second biggest search engine, processing more than 3 billion searches a month, second only to Google, which purchased YouTube in 2006 (Global Reach, 2020).

- **Instagram:** This is a photo- and video-sharing platform owned by Facebook. Like Twitter, the use of hashtags (#) is common on Instagram to help aggregate content based on specific topics.

- **Twitter:** Twitter is an online news and social networking platform where users can post updates and interact with messages known as tweets. Tweets are restricted to 280 characters to keep messages short and succinct. Hashtags (#) are used in front of a word or phrase to help aggregate content based on specific topics.

- **Google My Business:** This is a free local business listing service provided by Google to display your business or organization's information on Google maps and in searches. Google My Business listings quickly and easily provide information such as hours, phones numbers, addresses, photos, and reviews while also allowing customers to interact by guiding them to the website, inviting them to call, and more.

- **LinkedIn:** LinkedIn is a social network for professionals that is similar to Facebook but more focused on industry and professional news.

- **Pinterest:** Pinterest is a social media platform described as a "visual discovery engine" where users may search for a range of topics and ideas and save them to virtual "pin boards."

- **Reddit:** This is a website that aggregates news, provides internet content ratings, and allows for discussion among users. Members of this network may submit content including links, text, and images to the website that other members may "vote up" if they feel it contributes to a conversation or "down vote" if they feel it isn't of value or is off-topic.

- **Yelp:** This local search service is designed to help people find information about businesses and services in their area. Users may post reviews of businesses they have visited in order to help other users determine whether they want to patronize a given business.

- **Snapchat:** This social networking app allows users to capture and edit pictures and videos with special filters and share them with family and friends. Geofilters can be uploaded by users who want to draw attention to a particular event or location.

- **TikTok:** This video-sharing platfom provides users the opportunities to create short videos from three seconds to one minute and three seconds in length. The app includes features such as background music, filters, and video editing tools to create content such as comedy, dance, and education. TikTok's users are primarily teens and young adults.

- **Word of mouth:** Word of mouth marketing takes place as consumers share their experiences with a specific business, organization, product, or service in conversation with others and is considered a form of free advertising.

  - **Strategic partnerships:** intentional actions taken to build relationships with people or organizations who share the same or a similar audience as your own

  - **Testimonials:** positive comments provided by customers as a way to endorse a particular business, product, or service

  - **Online reviews:** reviews of a business, product, or service created by customers and posted to online review boards such as Google My Business

  - **Customer surveys:** a manner of collecting feedback from an audience to measure how satisfied customers are with a business, product, or service

PRO TIP: Some people actually start off with planning out their tactics, but it really should be one of your last steps before you launch your marketing plan. If you've taken the time to learn about your audience, their pain points and needs, and where and how they consume information, it helps you create a more intentional plan and messaging strategy. This allows you to see what is resonating with your audience and to pivot quickly when you notice gaps or areas where your message isn't sticking.

Resources and Budget

You will always want to do more than your resources will allow. You need to take your available resources into account when you are developing your plan. Resources include your budget and your time, as well as your connections. Because community development can include more than just your organization, you will want to consider what tools and resources your partners have available as well.

PRO TIP: Your goal here is to be lazy! In this context, lazy means that you want to choose the tactics that will take the least amount of resources to produce the greatest results.

Schedule

When you are in planning mode building your marketing plan, it is very easy to grow your plan out of the context of your reality. The final step in building your marketing plan is to create a schedule of all of the elements that you want to include and map what this will look like over time. This is a good check-and-balance moment so that you are crafting a plan that is relevant to your organization and stage of growth. The schedule is there to start off your process but needs to be editable and flexible so that you are shifting your plans to achieve your results, not just check the boxes and stay busy.

PRO TIP: If you have great scheduling tools, use them. If not, a spreadsheet will do just fine.

Final Thoughts: Marketing with Intention

Putting so much effort into getting the word out about an event or your community is called being intentional with your marketing efforts; it entails thinking about what you want people to do with the message you're putting out into the world. When you market with intention, your message is more likely to resonate with your audience than if you just shoot from the hip, post a couple of messages on social media about it, and hope it connects with people. Developing a marketing plan for your community will take some time, but when you are this intentional with your efforts, you will set yourself up for better success. As you achieve your goals, you will realize the time and effort is worth the work.

Case Study
Greenville, South Carolina

Located in northwestern South Carolina, Greenville is a large and rapidly growing city with industries based primarily in agriculture and textiles from the 1880s until the 1960s, with some other support industries. Eventually, the textile industry began to shrink, and companies began closing and sending jobs overseas, causing the late 1980s into the early 1990s to be a particularly tough time for the local economy and job market.

Just before the textile industry began to decline in Greenville, nearby Spartanburg started recruiting European companies to relocate or expand their operations into the United States, allowing for the formation of strategic partnerships between upstate South Carolina communities and foreign companies looking to expand their operations into the United States. Michelin opened a plant in Spartanburg County in 1973, which helped kickstart a change for the entire upstate South Carolina region. During this time, leaders from the area also recruited BMW, which opened its first facility outside of Germany in Spartanburg. The successes of these companies have helped persuade other foreign companies to either relocate or expand into the upstate region.

As these events were taking place, Greenville's city leadership took note. Prior to the 1970s, downtown Greenville was not a place people wanted to go as there wasn't much to see or do, and the area didn't have a great reputation. The community marketing efforts had been very haphazard and unintentional and couldn't be distinguished from those of any other community in efforts to attract industry and workforce. However, then-mayor Max Heller saw great potential in revitalizing the downtown area into a place people would want to be.

The city's leadership team understood the valuable assets Greenville held as the textile industry left and leveraged them to brand the community to attract European companies to locate in the city. They were able to define three target audiences: the internal audience served by the city's leadership, the external audience of the counties where many in Greenville's workforce lived, and partners in the public and private sector who also wanted to see new growth in the area.

Greenville's leaders knew their city's history and what they wanted it to become, adopting the tagline *Downtown is Everybody's Neighborhood* to emphasize that Greenville is a place for everyone (Whitworth & Neal, n.d.). They were able to tell their story in a way that made others realize their own potential for success in the area because they believed that Greenville could be a place where businesses would thrive and people would enjoy visiting. The cooperation that already existed among the public and private sectors positioned Greenville in a way that helped external audiences see their own potential; the leadership was able to communicate a strong desire to see businesses succeed there. A major contributing factor in the city's success was the strategic partnerships the city had already been building, which was one of its main marketing strategies in a pre-social media world.

As leaders in Greenville worked to attract new businesses, they understood the need for making the city an attractive place to live to retain and recruit a great workforce. This realization led to a new level of branding to residents and started with the vision to redevelop the downtown area. Drawing on the city's welcoming spirit and Southern hospitality, Greenville's brand personality, voice, and identity began to unfold. People started connecting with the idea that this was their neighborhood and a place where they belonged. With assistance from other key community leaders, Heller's vision for the North Main area began to take shape. An Urban Development Action Grant was secured and paved the way for the development of the Hyatt Regency Greenville, a key piece of the city's revitalization efforts.

As the area continued to grow, more opportunities emerged for the public and private sectors to work in cooperation to bring new developments that would create more jobs and improve the quality of life for residents. One such example is the Peace Center for the Performing Arts, which opened in 1990 on the former site of three old factories—one used for building wagons in the Civil War, a textile plant constructed in the 1880s, and a building that had once housed Duke's Mayonnaise. Another noteworthy milestone in Greenville's growth was the development of the river area in the late 1990s and early 2000s, with Mayor Knox White playing an instrumental role in establishing Falls Park as well as bringing the popular Mast General Store and Fluor Field to downtown.

All of these efforts have helped position Greenville for long-term success. The city is attractive to businesses looking to relocate or expand their operations, as well as to current and new residents alike. A testament to this work is the city's #10 ranking in Livability.com's 2019 Top 100 Best Places to Live list. Contributing factors to this ranking included Greenville's Housing Affordability Index of 92, 3.5% unemployment rate, quality healthcare options, and the vast array of experiences the city has to offer to those who live and work in the area.

In addition, the successes of relocated companies such as Michelin, BMW, Bosch, and GE, the city's proximity to other major hubs in the southeast and the Port of Charleston, a workforce prime for textiles and manufacturing, and the overall welcoming and cooperative spirit, have helped draw in interest from other major brands, including Amazon for its HQ2 project (HQ2 was eventually awarded to Crystal City, Arlington, Virginia). With a great regional airport, I-26 and I-85 nearby, and connection to the inland port in Greer plus the Port of Charleston deepening project expected to be complete by 2021, Greenville and the rest of the upstate region are prime for growth and continually working to improve its assets for all who live and work in the area.

Sources: Author conversations with John Lummus, President and CEO of Upstate South Carolina Alliance; Whitworth & Neal, n.d.

References

Carr, S. (2020, April 9). How many ads do we see a day in 2020? *PPC Protect.* https://ppcprotect.com/how-many-ads-do-we-see-a-day/.

Collins, J. & Portas, J.I. (1994) *Built to last. Successful habits of visionary companies.* William Collins.

Dibb, A. (2018). *The 1-page marketing plan: Get new customers, make more money, and stand out from the crowd.* Successwise.

Hyatt, M. (2018). *Your best year ever: A 5-step plan for achieving your most important goals.* Baker Books.

Jiwa, B. (2014, February 3). *Difference: The one-page method for reimagining your business and reinventing your marketing.* The Story of Telling Press.

Strategy. (n.d.). *Merriam-Webster.* (Online Dictionary). https://www.merriam-webster.com/dictionary/strategy.

Public Relations Society of America. (n.d.). *Public relations.* http://www.prsa.org/about/all-about-pr

Whitworth, N. & Neal, M. (n.d.). *How Greenville, South Carolina, brought downtown back: A case study in 30 years of successful public/private collaboration.* Save Our Gateways to Historic Brunswick & The Golden Isles of Georgia. http://saveourgateways.com/HowGreenville.php

Measuring Community Progress

Rhonda Phillips, PhD, FAICP

Measuring progress in community and economic development shows local citizens how their efforts in moving the community forward are paying off. Demonstrating progress and celebrating good news encourages individuals and organizations in the community to work harder and plan more effectively. Learn about different categories of community indicators—social, political, economic—and various measures within each specific group. Learn also how to set up and monitor these community indicators and other best practices and benchmarking to aid measuring progress.

Learning Outcomes

- Participants will learn strategies for documenting impact.

- Participants will be able to track short-term and long-term outcomes, data, and other stories that show a return on investment for the resources expended.

Achieving what a community wants for its goals and desired outcomes takes much dedicated work and time. There are many steps in the community development process, with changes and challenges emerging throughout. And just as with financial investments, past performances are not necessarily indicative of future results. In other words, an approach may have worked well in the past but may not be suitable for addressing current issues. Or another community may have had great success with a new program or policy, but given varying conditions inherent in each place, it may not be feasible for your community. The "bandwagon effect" can only take us so far with trying to replicate successes in other places in our own efforts.

As you might guess from the title of this chapter, there are ways to deal with ambiguity and many unknowns in trying to push communities forward in their development trajectories. By measuring progress, we can have a better sense of what works and what doesn't, and how best to approach solving challenges and issues to get to where we want to be in our communities. But to measure progress, we have to *evaluate*. Evaluation methods and processes have been around for a long time, in myriad contexts. It is the *systematic determination of the value or quality of a process, program, system, strategy, product, or service* (Davidson, 2005). It aids communities in developing, evolving, implementing, and improving their efforts. And every time something new is tried? Evaluation can help consider the value of any policy, strategy, program, process or system (Davidson, 2005).

Within community development (CD), evaluation is extremely relevant and needed "because citizens' quality of life is affected by such policies, programs, strategies, etc. If the impact and outcomes have not been soundly evaluated, can it be said that one approach is better than another or has a more positive influence" (Phillips & Pittman, 2015, p. 346)? Identifying what works is key, especially for justifying resources used in CD, whether in the public, private, or nonprofit and civic sectors. Knowing the impact and outcomes of investments is beneficial to many aspects of the CD process. This chapter provides an overview and context of measuring progress, beginning with some key foundational issues and aspects in the next section. This is followed by approaches to measuring progress; case studies conclude the chapter, providing suggestions and examples of tracking short- and long-term outcomes, data and stories to support measuring progress.

The Context of Measuring Progress

There is nothing easy or quick about CD at any level—whether local, regional, national, or multinational in scope. It is a very hard task to determine if the ends (outcomes) are reflected in estimates of the worth of the means (efforts, investments, etc.). Managi and Kumar (2018) explain that it is especially difficult because the ends include the well-being of future persons as well as the state of our environments as changed by use over time. They point out that "the reasoning involved in bringing the interests of people in the distant future into decisions over the deployment of today" is hard terrain to navigate. Of course, the timelines for consideration vary—for those more concerned with long-term sustainability, these considerations will weigh more heavily in decision making. But regardless of timeline, each community has to reflect on the future impacts of actions taken today. Indeed, the rise of sustainability and resilience as key features in CD is also embedded within evaluation not only for communities but also private companies (the rise of socially responsible businesses) and the public and civic sectors with more demands for accountability and transparency of decision making.

The Really Big Picture

Questions around sustainability and resilience abound at every level. At the multinational to the local levels, there is much discussion about whether or not current measures of progress used since the conclusion of World War II are best. Gross Domestic Product (GDP) is most commonly used; attempts to go beyond this utilitarian economic measure incorporate more reflections of overall social well-being. GDP has many uses; its original intention is to measure the value added in an economy within a specific time period. A 2009 report by Joseph Stiglitz and others that gained much attention on the topic of measures beyond those currently used suggested that GDP faces three challenges: conventional problems, quality-of-life aspects, and sustainability issues (Managi, 2018, p. 3).

These efforts aren't new—since the advent in 1987 of the Brundtland Commission's Report, *Our Common Future*, more attention has been called to sustainable development, defined in this report along with principles that have guided subsequent action (United Nations Sustainable Development, 2020a). We can see the inclusion of some of these thoughts about sustainability and quality of life in evaluation approaches including the triple bottom line of the *three e's*—economic, environmental, and equity (some refer to equity as social/cultural aspects)—or *three p's*—people, planet, and profit (Slaper & Hall, 2011). Much work has been done while pursuing the United Nation's Sustainability Goals introduced in 2015 (United Nations Sustainable Development, 2020b). These goals have influenced work from local to multinational levels across the three dimensions of economic, environmental, and equity aspects of life, and this is why we mention it. It's highly likely some of the same things you're working on in your community are reflected in some of these goals and approaches across the globe.

As expected, ongoing debates and suggested uses include measuring other dimensions of people's experiences such as well-being, happiness (flourishing), and quality of life. Community indicators, which will be discussed later in this chapter, "offer an opportunity to go beyond a standard economic indicator, such as gross domestic product, to fully assess well-being" (Phillips, 2003, p. 25). Quality of life, most simply described, is how individuals are experiencing life. The World Health Organization defines quality of life as "individuals' perceptions of their position in life in the context of the culture and value systems in which they live and in relation to their goals, expectations, standards and concerns" (Phillips, 2003, p. 1).

Community Well-being

Because well-being is a trending topic and has relevance for measuring progress, let's explore this more. In the context of where we live, *community well-being* is a wide-ranging concept encompassing multiple dimensions that are related to people and their communities. It includes "comprehensive and integrated concepts developed by synthesizing research constructs related to residents' perceptions of the community, residents' needs fulfillment, observable community conditions, and the social and cultural context of the community" (Sung & Phillips 2016). In other words, community well-being has many dimensions to it—whether social, economic, or environmental in nature. Types of governance structure, for example, as well as the physical environment—and certainly the needs and desires of a community's residents—impact well-being. As explained by Phillips & Wong (2017):

> Community well-being can also be thought of as an overarching concept with related conceptions such as happiness, quality of life, and community development often being mentioned jointly or interchangeably. These concepts are highly related yet different, given the scale or context. For example, happiness is often thought of as an individual state of being, although there are attempts of finding the collective happiness of communities, regions, or even countries (p. xxix).

While this may seem far afield from the practice and application of community development at the local level, it's important to remember the core foundational principle of CD: to improve people's conditions in the built, social, environmental, and economic dimensions where we live. It includes guiding practices such as social capacity building as well as participatory and inclusive processes for realizing desired outcomes. CD is very often part of public policy and governance as well as city and regional planning practice. So how does community well-being differ from community development? Most often, the difference is found in that CD is focused on taking action in the public, social, and private sectors to achieve desirable goals while community well-being can be used for assessing states of being and not necessarily taking action (Sung and Phillips, 2016).

Why Measure Progress?

Interest continues to grow in making improvements in local level decision making regarding community development projects, processes, and investments; this includes documenting outcomes (Blanke & Walzer, 2013). This growing interest in better measurement practices is not only about a specific program—it is driven by the need to monitor overall conditions and explore ways to make good decisions and investments about a whole host of things that influence communities (p. 535).

It is one thing to say we want to measure progress and a different thing to actually do it. It is not easy but rather quite challenging to measure outcomes in the public and nonprofit sectors, because it requires considering many aspects of activities, inputs and outputs, and impacts that may require much data collection (W.K. Kellogg Foundation, 2017; Walzer, Leonard & Emery, 2013). Small towns and cities or neighborhoods may find it especially challenging, but the good news is that improvements have been made in constructing and documenting measurement practices, such as those by the Community Indicators Consortium (CIC, 2020). But measure, analyze, and assess we must, because many aspects of achieving success in CD depend upon it, not the least of which is to continue securing sources of funding to carry out programs and services as well as influence public policy with evidenced-based shared information. It is important to remember to implement evaluation approaches that can be easily and feasibly used, or the effort is wasted. Perhaps the only good evaluation is one that can be done and subsequently used.

Approaches to Measuring Progress

There are many ways to measure progress using a variety of evaluation techniques. This chapter focuses on approaches that are applicable and doable, regardless of budget or staffing constraints. For the purposes of CD, here are a few of the more relevant: benchmarking and best practices and community indicators. First, let's consider some of the approaches used more broadly. Generally, there is a cycle to evaluation that ties deeply to visioning, planning, and implementation. A way to think about this is as a cycle, starting with identifying or refining goals, vision, mission and actions. Here is one such example, termed the Measuring, Monitoring, Tracking and Reporting (MMTR) cycle:

• Establishing goals, vision, mission, and targets

• Determining benchmark data, year, and end year

• Assigning target champions

• Aligning the targets with budget/fiscal plans

• Monitoring and tracking

• Measuring using qualitative and quantitative data

• Reporting and disseminating results and progress update (Alibašić, 2018, p. 47)

This is somewhat similar to planning for community development at the local level, with the exception that in the latter, more participation and inclusion of residents and stakeholders would be needed in the decision-making process. The point is that at the local level, planning processes typically include assessment or evaluation at some stage in the cycle; those communities that skip over this critical component of the development process may not achieve what they set out to do. Blanke and Walzer (2015) assert that creating a feedback loop connecting changes in key measures to resulting policy approaches or program adjustments is one of the *essential components* in the development process.

Benchmarking and Best Practices

All communities face their own unique situations and challenges. At the same time, some common issues cut across different places, and this is why benchmarking and best practices can be of value. Simply put, benchmarking is determining peers to compare your community to and seeing where your community measures up to the others. It can be a regional peer, national, or beyond; it really depends on what is going to be compared. Regional, national or international standards can be used (such as the case in sustainability), or the local area can determine what they want to compare and use as benchmarks (for example, environmental benchmarks such as reducing landfill waste). Best practices are just as they sound—a successful approach to achieving a goal that has been "tried and tested" by other communities and can serve as examples or models of what can be done in your own community.

Where to start with benchmarking and best practices as part of measuring your community's progress towards goals? First, find general ideas and information for benchmarking and best practices from which to learn. Sometimes this is easy—we may often hear of successes in other communities through the media or professional associations. Sources for this type of information include utility companies with active economic and community development programs; universities with development centers; local, regional, or state departments of development; and regional or national professional associations such as the Southern Economic Development Council or the Community Development Council. Publications that focus on development will also have best practices examples featured.

After an information scan is conducted, a few more steps remain to conduct a best practices/benchmarking study. Phillips and Pittman (2015) provide the following guidance:

1. Identify the topic. The more specific and definable the better.

2. Identify the communities or areas with which you want to be compared. Usually four to six communities are sufficient for best practices comparisons. Often, the comparison communities are of similar size and situation. However, some prefer to benchmark themselves against exemplary communities they hope to emulate.

3. Call the appropriate representative(s) from the comparison communities and explain the process. Determine whether the participants prefer to remain anonymous or not. Decide whether you will share the results with the participants in return for their cooperation.

4. Develop a survey form and decide is it is going to be administered by telephone or in-person conversation, or via internet or otherwise. If possible, travel to the comparison communities to obtain the best results (and observations).

5. Administer the best practices/benchmarking survey and collate the results. Compare your community against the others on all questions and analyze how yours is different or alike. Based on the survey results, develop program recommendations.

Benchmarking and best practices are a relatively easy way to find examples and ideas for moving forward in your own community. While they won't provide all the answers, it is a start to help with the visioning process, asking questions such as, "What do we want to be like in a year, in three or five years or longer?" "How can we take action today to help work towards our goals?" and so on. All of us have visited or lived in places that have been successful in various aspects of community development; learning from them is a natural way to move forward. At the same time, each community needs to tailor their own approaches to suit them and reflect what is desired for the future.

Community Indicators

Community indicators are essentially data points that, when combined, generate a picture of what is happening in a local system (Phillips, 2003). When used as an evaluation system or approach, they hold much promise for combining ongoing evaluation into overall development efforts. Indicator systems can be quite elaborate and run for many years, or be more targeted for specific, time-delineated purposes. In this chapter, let's focus on indicators that can be identified or created and used in a way that is both feasible and useful without extensive investment of time and resources. This becomes easier when the purpose of indicators is thought of as follows:

> The goal is to elicit participation from community residents and other organizations to identify and construct indicators to influence policy outcomes in the public sector (Phillips, 2003, p. 14).

In other words, the idea is to use indicators to get to where the community wants to be both now and in the future via policies and the programs, investments, and resources that are used to implement them. Here's an example—when the residents of Seattle, Washington noticed that the wild salmon weren't coming back as much as in the past to spawn in the rivers, they got really concerned and interested in monitoring environmental quality of the waterways. They developed indicators that directly influenced the city to respond with policies to protect the rivers with actions such as limiting runoff and other measures. This effort grew into a major indicator project encompassing economic and social/cultural issues; a nonprofit, Sustainable Seattle, was formed and became widely known. The project has closed after many years and positive outcomes on development processes in the city. The following lists a few of the indicators they used (and subsequently many other indicator projects used them as "best practices" examples). In addition to typical indicators like unemployment rates or housing affordability, they used indicators that provided deeper insight into conditions in the city. For example, distribution of personal income included aspects such as percentage of income spent on housing and related indicators to give an overview of that area; employment concentration would include aspects that show whether or not there is enough diversity in the economy.

- **Environmental:**
  Ecological health
  Soil erosion
  Air quality

- **Economy:**
  Distribution of personal income
  Employment concentration
  Community reinvestment

- **Health and community:**
  Voter participation
  Perceived quality of life
  Low birth-weight infants

Indicators can be thought of as gauges, providing insight into whether progress is being made or not towards goals that are decided upon, typically via a community planning visioning process. Having residents participate in identifying their values and priorities makes it easier to identify or create indicators. Budruk and Phillips (2011) provide the following that explains this context for indicators:

1. What makes community indicators any different from other measures? Their specialness lies in the ability to help build an integrative approach—considering impacts in not only economic terms, but also the social and environmental dimensions. It is the ability to build a system or framework on valid indicators that conveys its real usefulness. These systems can then be used to aid decision making and set priorities within organizations and communities.

2. Further, an indicator system reflects collective values of a community, and this is a powerful feature. If the process of identifying and implementing indicators is open and inclusive, i.e., if citizen and stakeholder participation are embedded in the process, then the system will reflect collective values. Typically, decisions made on the basis of collective values receive more widespread support since collective values imply that goals or targets are more widely agreed upon.

3. Finally, indicators' systems or frameworks represent a more comprehensive evaluation tool. Since these systems can be integrated into community development planning for an overall community or region's planning, it makes evaluation easier (pp. 2–4).

Next, let's explore how to identify or create indicators by exploring some cases. We will consider the processes they used which can provide insight into ideas for your own community.

Case Studies

Typically, a core set of indicators will be identified for a community to use; this is usually between 20 to 50 individual indicators, although some like to create composite indicators with a few metrics for each. The example above, identifying some of those Seattle used, includes composite indicators (combining several individual indicators to paint a picture of the impact). Weights can be assigned too, especially if there are some indicators that are viewed as higher priority. It usually takes a few months to identify and design a basic community indicator system. Ideally, the system will be updated over time and remain in place long enough to monitor community change. You will note that some indicator systems start off with a bang with funding and fanfare and then dissipate over time. This is due to a few reasons: the original impetus for creating them is resolved (such as a major employer pulling out or a specific environmental challenge) or the system was complex and required more resources than could be provided over time. You will also see many sponsors for indicator systems too, this is because the sources of data are often not centralized and require participation by multiple partners. This section provides a few types of examples of community indicator projects or systems: (1) a city-based indicator project embedded within other public policies; (2) a partnership-based model; and (3) a specific issue indicator project. The first is that of Burlington, Vermont (population 43,000) that uses indicators as part of their planning process. The second is from Spartanburg County, South Carolina (population 300,000) and illustrates a system that has many partners from both the public and private sectors. The third is a framework that is provided to consider a specific issue—in this case, historic preservation.

Case Study
Burlington, Vermont: A Community Indicator System Embedded Within Public Sector Planning

This small city on the shores of Lake Champlain near the Canadian border has long been concerned with sustainability issues. Beginning in 2000, the city decided to respond to residents' requests with the Legacy Project Action Plan, providing a blueprint for environmental, economic, social, and cultural health over the long term. To do so, they embedded the Legacy Project within their comprehensive plans so that goals and indicators could be monitored and acknowledged throughout time as decisions were made. Five major themes emerged from their participation processes and updated periodically with the plans:

- maintain Burlington as a regional population, government, cultural, and economic center, matching job growth and family incomes

- improve quality of life in neighborhoods

- increase participation in public decision making

- provide youth with high-quality education and social supports and lifelong learning opportunities for all

- preserve environmental health (City of Burlington, 2000).

These five areas represent the values that residents prioritize. Tying goals to actions and indicators to monitor progress towards those goals is a very efficient and clear-cut approach. It doesn't allow for ambiguity that is sometimes present when indicators are not tied to specific actions or embedded within policies and plans at the local governance level. Anyone can quickly see if progress is being made or not with this type of scenario when data are shared and transparent. Updates are made periodically; now the following areas are assigned goals, actions, and indicators: diversity and equity; economy; education and lifelong learning; environment; governance; neighborhoods; and transportation (City of Burlington, 2013).

Here's how the city actualizes these desired themes through action. First, they identified multiple goals that reflect the themes. After goal identification based on a community participatory process, actions were assigned to each. Finally, major indicators are used to gauge progress. For our example, let's use economic self-reliance with its goal statement, actions, and indicators.

Economic Self Reliance

Goal: In 2030, Burlington has become more self-reliant through local ownership, control, and maximum use and reinvestment of local resources.

A sustainable economy requires a high degree of self-reliance and a diverse mix of businesses in a dynamic environment. Participants in the Legacy Project have spoken repeatedly of the need for increased local ownership of and support for local businesses. They have also called for the city and its people to make maximum use of local resources for basic needs. This will anchor the local economy, which will need to successfully navigate the open waters of the global economy in years to come. Burlington has a strong base and tradition of local ownership and self-reliance upon which to build. The Burlington Electric Department reports that there are 2,500 businesses within the city and 11 percent of all adults are self-employed. The Intervale (a farm incubator located on a former brownfield inside the city limits) is home to nine agricultural businesses, seven vegetable farms, a $400,000 composting project, and the wood-fired McNeil electrical generating station.

Priority Actions:

- Develop and implement additional incentives and technical support to create a dynamic business mix. Create new businesses, livable-wage job opportunities, and economic development by providing goods and services locally.

- Support micro- and small business development, including women- and minority-owned enterprises.

- Increase production and marketing of agricultural products in the Intervale and support the distribution and consumption of locally produced foods through public and farmer's markets, a "food train," community gardens, and community supported agriculture (CSA).

- Develop an "Eco-Park" in the Intervale to create well-paying jobs tied to local agriculture and natural resources.

- Develop more affordable commercial and incubator spaces downtown and in other designated areas throughout the city.

Other Actions:

1. Combine the purchasing power of major institutions in the city (including the University of Vermont, Fletcher Allen Healthcare, and the City of Burlington) to support businesses that will direct dollars to the local economy.

2. Encourage individuals, businesses, and organizations to invest savings in local financial institutions that reinvest funds directly back into the community. Promote active community reinvestment among all local banks and financial institutions.

3. Provide creative financing and affordable capital for business growth through public/private partnerships.

Measuring Progress: Indicators to Watch

- Number of Burlington business startups and closings
- Businesses per sector by size

(Later, other indicators such as number of employee-owned businesses or non-profit organizations activities began to be used,)

Source: https://www.burlingtonvt.gov/Sustainability/Legacy-Action-Plan

Case Study

A Partnership Community-wide System: Spartanburg, South Carolina

This model is seen throughout the U.S. and Canada as a way to have a strong, cross-sector presence with indicators to call attention to issues as well as encourage action. Typically, it is a nonprofit organization that coordinates and houses the indicator project of this larger-scale type. **The Spartanburg Community Indicators Project** gathers and compiles a variety of data across seven indicator areas. Periodic updates and reports are released, and the intention is to engage "the community in dialogue and strategy that leads to positive change in Spartanburg County, South Carolina. The project facilitates organizations and individuals as they actively promote civic prosperity by using community indicator data to inform and guide their progress" (Spartanburg Community Indicators Project, 2020).

Partnerships are a key feature of this type of indicator system, where funding comes from a variety of sources. For this project, it represents a collaboration of the following organizations: the Spartanburg County Foundation; United Way of the Piedmont; Spartanburg County; University of South Carolina Upstate; Spartanburg Regional Foundation; and Spartanburg Area Chamber of Commerce.

Here is the listing of some of their areas, along with the goal statement and indicators for each.

Area: Civic Health

Indicator Area Leader: Spartanburg County Public Libraries

Goal: Our citizens will have access to opportunities for civic engagement that promote community well-being and an enriched quality of life.

Indicators:

- Voter Turnout: scytl.us, scvotes.org
- Percentage attendance in public meetings: Corporation for National and Community Service
- Number of volunteer hours: Corporation for National and Community Service
- Volunteer rate: Corporation for National and Community Service
- Percentage donating more than $25: Corporation for National and Community Service

Area: Economy

Indicator Area Leader: Spartanburg Area Chamber of Commerce

Goal: Our citizens will have access to living wage jobs and our communities will be economically viable.

Indicators:

- Household Income, *source: United States Census Bureau*
- Median Worker Earnings, 16+, *source: United States Census Bureau*
- Per Capita Income, *source: United States Census Bureau*
- Poverty, *source: United States Census Bureau*
- Unemployment Rates, *source: SC Works*
- Gross Sales, *source: South Carolina Department of Revenue and Taxation*
- Job Losses, *source: Appalachian Council of Governments*
- Worker Commuter Patterns, *source: United States Census Bureau*
- Employment & Wages, *source: Appalachian Council of Governments*

Area: Education

Indicator Area Leader: Spartanburg Academic Movement

Goal: Our children will excel academically and our citizens will demonstrate high levels of baccalaureate degree attainment, rendering Spartanburg the best educated county in the state.

Indicators:

- Educational Attainment, population 25+, *source: United States Census Bureau*
- High School Graduation Rates, 4-year, *source: South Carolina Department of Education*
- 3rd Grade ELA (English) Proficiency Rates, *source: South Carolina Department of Education*
- 8th Grade Math Proficiency Rates, *source: South Carolina Department of Education*
- 3k and 4k Enrollment Rates, *source: South Carolina Department of Education and United States Census Bureau*

Area: Natural Environment

Indicator Area Leader: Natural Environment Coalition

Goal: Our citizens will manage our natural resources in a way that will support current and future generations.

Indicators:

- Historic Ozone Values: South Carolina Department of Health and Environmental Control
- List of Impaired Water Bodies: South Carolina Department of Health and Environmental Control
- Existing Land Use: Spartanburg Comprehensive Plan
- Rare, Threatened, and Endangered Species: South Carolina Department of Natural Resources

Area: Public Health

Indicator Area Leader: The Road to Better Health

Goal: Our citizens will be increasingly healthy, demonstrating decreasing incidence and prevalence of health risk factors and poor health outcomes.

Indicators:

- Infant Mortality Rates, *source: South Carolina Department of Health and Environmental Control*
- Low Birthweight, *source: South Carolina Department of Health and Environmental Control*
- Per Capita Income, *source: United States Census Bureau*
- Prenatal Care, *source: South Carolina Department of Health and Environmental Control*
- Teen Birth Rates, *source: South Carolina Department of Health and Environmental Control*
- Emergency Department Visits, *source: South Carolina Revenue and Fiscal Affairs*

Area: Social Environment

Indicator Area Leader: Social Environment Coalition

Goal: Our community will be characterized by stable families, low crime, affordable housing and access to opportunity.

Indicators:

- Violent Crime: SLED
- Juvenile Data: South Carolina Department of Juvenile Justice
- Live Births to Single Mothers with Less than HS Education: Annie E. Casey Kids Count Data Center
- Live Births to Single Mothers: Annie E. Casey Kids Count Data Center
- Children in Foster Care: South Carolina Department of Social Services
- Child Neglect and Abuse: Annie E. Casey Kids Count Data Center

Source: Spartanburg County Community Indicators Project, www.strategicspartanburg.org/

Case Study
Specific Issue Indicator Framework: Historic Preservation

This is a bit of a different example, one that is designed for a specific issue or area to gauge. In this case, it is about historic preservation in a community or neighborhood. It is approached in a different way than wide-scale indicator projects, such as the example of Spartanburg above. Dealing with very specific measures and goals, the indicators presented in the following framework are typical of what could be used in a historic district. Of course, each community may have different aspects they want to monitor in a designated area, such as percentage of owner-occupied homes in the district. Given the rise of newer models of short-term rentals, such as Airbnb, indicators to gauge activity levels of tourists may be needed.

Four categories of indicators are presented, along with listings of the types of data that could be used in each. The four categories reflect various issue areas: gauging (related to type and amount, perceptions and values); protecting (ordinances and regulations); enhancing (partnerships and incentives); and interfacing (uses). The following presents a listing of the indicators. More information on the rationale for selection, definitions, and dimensions is presented by Phillips and Stein (2011).

Note that this type of approach can be used for other specific purposes too, not only a historic neighborhood but also for other applications. This may include applications for a development district, a special use area, or other projects that have a defined purpose or goal. It can also be used for a program that is not necessarily physical but policy- or action-oriented, such as education or collaborative efforts.

Indicators Framework for a Historic District

Types of Indicators

A. Gauging

Historic fabric

Districts, structures, landmarks

Distressed historic neighborhoods

Rehabilitation/certified tax credits

Assessed property value trends

Historic district/property reinvestment

Amount and type locally-owned businesses

Sense of place/identification with place/attachment to place

B. Protecting

Historic preservation element/plan and integration with community planning

Design guidelines

Historic preservation commission

Preservation ordinances

Historic preservation survey

Historic preservation staff

Certificates and enforcement actions

C. Enhancing

Participation in Main Street or other nationally sponsored programs

Certified Local Government status or other certification programs

Participation in other state/federal programs

Number and type of historic preservation nonprofit organizations

Neighborhood participation

Civic/museum partnerships Incentive programs

Gentrification—programs to prevent

D. Interfacing

- Use and access by citizens—internal, external, visible, cost
- Housing affordability and percent affordable historic houses
- Business use and types
- Community draw factors
- Community use factors
- Heritage/cultural interactions and skills

Source: Phillips & Stein, 2011, p. 6.

Moving Forward

As mentioned in a prior section, many available resources address community development best practices or benchmarking examples from around the U.S. and beyond. Of course, ideas from other places are great to build on while taking into account the needs and desires of your own community. Being able to use benchmarks and best-practice comparisons enables a community to conduct a timely and affordable evaluation or measure of progress achievement fairly readily.

Community indicators can also be used, especially if tied to a visioning or planning process to create or identify indicators that really reflect community values. Indicators are very useful for gauging progress towards goals or alerting a community of issues or challenges that need attention. To recap, a major goal of using community indicators is to influence public policy so that resources and investments can be channeled where needed most. There are also many sources of indicator systems and applications. One of the best sources, mentioned earlier, is that of the Community Indicators Consortium that provides a list of hundreds of projects. Most public and nonprofit indicator projects are readily available for viewing via the internet.

Likewise, there are many readily available sources for evaluation and other approaches that can be used to gauge and understand how actions impact outcomes. One example is that of the Community Toolkit that provides a comprehensive workbook on various aspects of evaluation ("Evaluating Community Programs and Initiatives," 2020). Measuring progress is one of the most essential aspects of community development; wishing you much success in your efforts to do so!

References

Alibašić, H. (2018). *Sustainability and resilience planning for local governments: The quadruple bottom line strategy*. Springer.

Blanke, A.S. & Walzer, N. (2013). Measuring community development: What have we learned? *Community Development, 44*(5), 534–550. https://doi.org/10.1080/15575330.2013.852595

Budruk, M. & Phillips, R. (2011). *Quality-of-life community indicators for parks, recreation and tourism management*. Springer.

City of Burlington, Vermont. (2000). *Legacy action plan*. https://www.burlingtonvt.gov/sites/default/files/CEDO/Legacy_Project/Legacy%20Action%20Plan.pdf.

City of Burlington, Vermont. (2013). *Burlington legacy project*. https://www.burlingtonvt.gov/sites/default/files/uploadedfiles/BurlingtonVTgov/Departments/Legacy/The_Legacy_Plan/Legacy%20Action%20Plan%20Update-all%206%20sectors%201-31-13.pdf.

Community Indicators Consortium (CIC). (2020). *Sources of data available for U.S. community indicator projects*. https://communityindicators.net/research/sources-of-data-available-for-u-s-community-indicators-projects/

Davidson, E.J. (2005). *Evaluation methodology basics*. Sage.

Evaluating community programs and initiatives. (2020). In *Community Tool Box*. Center for Community Health and Development, University of Kansas. https://ctb.ku.edu/en/evaluating-community-programs-and-initiatives.

Managi, S. & Kumar, P. (2018). *Inclusive wealth report 2018*. (1st ed). Routledge.

Managi, S. (2018). Accounting for the inclusive wealth of nations. In S. Managi & P, Kumar (Eds.). (2018). *Inclusive wealth report 2018* (pp. 3–52). Routledge.

Maurice, J. (2016). Measuring progress towards the SDGs: A new vital science. *The Lancet*. 388 (10053), 1455–1458.

Organization for Economic Cooperation and Development (OECD). (2008). *Statistics, knowledge and policy 2007: Measuring and fostering the progress of societies*. OECD Publishing.

Phillips, R. (2003). *Community Indicators*. Planning Advisory Service Report No. 517. American Planning Association.

Phillips, R. & Pittman, R. (2015). *Introduction to community development*. (2nd ed.). Routledge.

Phillips, R. & Stein, J. (2011). An indicator framework for linking historic preservation and community economic development. *Social Indicators Research* 113, 1–15.

Phillips, R. & Wong, C. (2017). *Handbook of community well-being research*. Springer.

Slaper, T. & Hall, T. (2011). The triple bottom line: What is IT and how does it work? *Indiana Business Review*, 83(1), 4–8.

Spartanburg Community Indicators Project. (2020). *Strategic Spartanburg*. https://www.strategicspartanburg.org

Sung, H. & Phillips, R. (2016). Conceptualizing a community well-being and theory construct. In S.J. Lee, Y. Kim & R. Phillips (Eds.). (2016). *Social Factors and Community Well-Being* (pp. 1–12). Springer.

United Nations Sustainable Development. (2020a). *Report of the world commission on environment and development: Our common future*. https://sustainabledevelopment.un.org/milestones/wced.

United Nations Sustainable Development. (2020b). *Sustainable development goals*. https://www.un.org/sustainabledevelopment/sustainable-development-goals/

Walzer, N., Leonard, J. & Emery, M. (2013) Overview of innovative measurement and evaluation issue. *Community Development, (44)*5, 529–533. https://doi.org/10.1080/15575330.2013.852596

W.K. Kellogg Foundation (2017). *The step-by-step guide to evaluation*. https://www.wkkf.org/resource-directory/resources/2017/11/the-step-by-step-guide-to-evaluation--how-to-become-savvy-evaluation-consumers

Workforce Planning and Development

Courtney Taylor, PhD, PCED & Heather Annulis, PhD, CPLP

A community's human capital is one of its most valuable assets. Communities and states must focus on developing the skill levels of their resident workforce or risk becoming noncompetitive in the global economy or losing jobs to other states. This program addresses one of the most significant challenges facing state and local governments across America—workforce planning, development, and management during an era of reduced budgets, growing expectations, and escalating demand. The program provides a comprehensive view of the workforce development pipeline, resources, and potential partners, and provides participants with strategies to engage local partners to ensure a pipeline of talent exists in the local community.

Learning Outcomes

- Participants will review the various components of workforce development and examine the relationships between workforce development, urbanization, and education.

- Participants will understand how workforce development and regional laborsheds impact the economic development process.

- Participants will study the effects of population shifts and evolving technology on workforce development initiatives.

In the early part of the 21st century, economic development projects centered on physical infrastructure within the United States. While physical infrastructure continues as a vital element of a community's overall quality of life, the ability to compete for new and expanding business and industry investments allows a community to prosper and overtake others economically. Additionally, a community's human capital often serves as the defining success factor (Benhabib & Spiegel, 1994). Policymakers, researchers, and practitioners call for increased efforts to not only increase and improve training and education efforts but also to align workforce and economic development activities with investments at the local level for more effective use of scarce resources (Conway, 2011).

The U.S. is experiencing a slower population growth rate than in previous decades, further complicated by a lower immigration rate. While fewer jobs exist, so do fewer people. Luckily, many new economic development projects are physical capital intensive; thus, they do not require as many workers as employers did a decade ago. Workers, however, must possess a greater skill level than in decades past, as many industries rely heavily on technology. There has arguably never been a better time to enhance local workforce development efforts to ensure a community's human capital can compete with the national and international workforce.

Workforce development is an essential element of community economic development. The definition of *workforce development* provided by Blum and Shepelwich (2017) is most relevant to those using this text: "Workforce development consists of a range of strategies to develop talent and skills, connect employers and workers, and facilitate career mobility" (p. 4). *Talent development* is also known as *human capital development*, and "at the individual level, human capital consists of the characteristics possessed by an individual that can yield positive outcomes for that individual while at the unit level, human capital can refer to the aggregate accumulation of individual human capital that can be combined in a way that creates value for the unit" (Wright & McMahan, 2011).

In other words, developing a community's human capital through workforce development can have benefits for both the individual and the community. Investments in individual training allow employees to flourish economically and employers to improve their bottom line. Employers in the U.S. provide most of the job training, spending 8 to 10 times more than the public sector (Carnevale, Strohl & Gulish, 2015; Mikelson & Nightingale, 2004). This investment in human capital, however, is more likely to go to highly educated and highly paid employees—not the skilled workers that employers demand of their local workforce system. The public workforce system in the U.S. serves a small portion of America's 150 million workers. Still, it serves those who likely would not receive training and is an essential component of improving the workforce locally.

The public workforce system in the U.S. is a partnership between federal, state, and local governments with the mission of providing employment-related services to two groups: workers and employers. Ten federal government agencies fund the system that supports job training programs. The primary agencies include the U.S. Departments of Labor, Education, Health and Human Services, and Veterans Affairs. The programs these agencies support include those funded through the Workforce Innovation and Opportunity Act (WIOA), which serves adults, youth, dislocated workers, the underemployed, individuals with disabilities, individuals with low basic skills, and others depending on the region. Additional programs provide funding for job training and support services through other agencies such as Temporary Assistance for Needy Families (TANF), Veterans Vocational Rehabilitation and Employment, Supplemental Assistance Program Employment and Training, and Career and Technical Education.

The Wagner-Peyser Act (1933) provided funding for "the establishment and maintenance of a national system of public employment offices" (U.S. Department of Labor, n.d.). Today, more than 2,000 local American Job Centers offer free job search and matching services, as well as access to and funding for training programs and support services to assist those entering the labor market (Nightingale & Eyster, 2018). A key to ensuring success for future workforce development of students, dislocated workers, and incumbent workers includes understanding the job opportunities available in the region and the available education and training pathways that help build and enhance a comprehensive workforce pipeline.

Workforce Pipeline

Fully developing a region's human capital requires alignment of the public school system, community colleges, four-year colleges and universities, and the public workforce system. The public school system was designed prior to the Industrial Revolution for an agrarian society. Today, leaders must address weaknesses and gaps, specifically the middle skills gap, which refers to the lack of qualified talent available to fill jobs requiring more than a high school education but less than a four-year degree. These jobs—nursing, high-skill manufacturing, computer technology, and others—represent approximately 52% of the jobs in the U.S., while only 43% of the population is skilled (National Skills Coalition, 2020). This gap drives much of the workforce development conversation as technology enhancements force increased requirements for skills in many industries. Additionally, estimates project that many of the current workers will be eligible to retire within the next decade, leaving a shortage of workers. Efforts to further develop the activities, programs, and funding available to assist the next generation in finding their careers must be continued and coordinated.

The public education system in the U.S. consists of primary, secondary, postsecondary, and higher education institutions. Primary and secondary institutions are not specifically charged with training for specific job skills. Instead, the institutions are responsible for the overall education of the nation's youth and serve as the fundamental building block for tomorrow's human capital. Exposing young adults to broad career pathways falls within the purview of the public education system at all levels. In addition, many federal agencies and skills-related organizations champion efforts of career exploration for youth across the U.S. Career exploration while in primary and secondary schooling encourages youth to examine all options available upon high school completion.

Community colleges and four-year colleges and universities serve both the public workforce system and the public education system. Community colleges, designed to serve their local communities, provide increased access to higher education and collaborate with local employers to provide a pipeline of skilled and productive workers through degree and nondegree training programs. Four-year education institutions support human capital and workforce development efforts by increasing the share of college-educated workers, producing relevant research, and partnering with secondary and postsecondary institutions to create valuable programs and initiatives. Community colleges and universities must align with the secondary system and the public workforce system to address weaknesses and gaps.

Primary Education

Because basic education is the foundation upon which all future education and workforce skills are built, primary education should be included in the workforce development strategies of today. Additionally, primary education should serve as a place to begin career exploration for youth. Engaging students, instructors, and counselors in activities designed for early career exploration exposes students to careers and allows interaction with professionals in the workplace. Community economic development partners and local leaders should engage with students by coordinating efforts to bring partners to school campuses, thereby allowing students to engage with representatives of local organizations that they may not otherwise be familiar with. Partners can work with teachers to design games and activities, allowing younger age groups to explore basic skills. Just as giving a young child a firetruck or a stethoscope to play with encourages their creativity and exposure, bringing other potentially nontraditional occupations to their attention may excite them and lead them to professions otherwise undiscovered. As students move to secondary education, they should begin to explore broad career pathways.

Secondary Education

Secondary education is increasingly targeted in workforce pipeline discussions as both a necessary partner and a source of concern. While institutions regularly expose high school students to four-year and two-year academic education opportunities, students often lack exposure to career and technical training available over a period of two years or less. Many secondary students graduate high school without any exposure to high-wage jobs within their region or to the educational pathways to those jobs. While many organizations strive to bring the opportunities to the forefront for students by ensuring students in secondary schools receive exposure to career pathways and related training and education programs, continued work must focus on increasing middle- and high-school students' understanding of the existing labor market and pathways to enter it. Additionally, secondary education providers must cease the singular pathway approach and work to provide students with many pathways, not treating any as better or worse than another.

States must reflect this in finding priorities as well. In recent years, efforts by the U.S. Departments of Labor, Education, and Health and Human Services encourage the use of career pathways in secondary education. Ensuring that programs align with the skill needs of industry—and that secondary schooling prepares individuals to be successful in a range of postsecondary pursuits, including academic degrees, career training, and registered apprenticeships—continues as a focus of these agencies.

To ensure success, secondary schools need local stakeholders to assist in connecting leaders to local partners such as community colleges, four-year institutions, career centers, and employers, among others. Community economic developers and local leaders can best assist secondary leaders by highlighting the full career pathway from high school through community college and on to work. Additionally, leaders should strive to ensure secondary programs guide students into relevant postsecondary programs. Partnerships between secondary and postsecondary entities remain vital in the career technical areas as training program costs can be expensive. These programs typically require extensive employer involvement. To ensure the best use of everyone's time, secondary and postsecondary leaders should combine efforts to engage employers. Community economic developers and leaders can assist by encouraging these actions and serving as a conduit to business and industry leaders.

Secondary and postsecondary institutions engage with each other in various ways—through dual enrollment, for example. Dual enrollment provides participants the opportunity to take college-level courses while still in high school. Dual enrollment provides many benefits, including:

- helping students shorten completion time of postsecondary studies by gaining credits early;

- saving students money through often discounted offerings;

- allowing students to pursue career technical courses (in areas providing Career and Technical Education—known as CTE—dual enrollment) while still in high school; and

- providing students of all socioeconomic backgrounds the opportunity to experience "college life" from the safety of a high school's infrastructure.

Many students, however, never receive encouragement to explore careers in order to determine occupations they may be interested in, nor are they encouraged to consider community college as a pathway.

Postsecondary Education

Postsecondary institutions have multiple missions. Community colleges are charged with both education and training, accomplished through various endeavors such as nondegree training programs, apprenticeships, academic education, career technical degree programs, and customized training for incumbent workers. Additionally, community colleges often serve as home to adult basic education programs designed to provide such resources as assistance with high school equivalency preparation and tests, ESL (English as a Second Language) training programs, and tutoring for basic skills. Providing a complete list of their activities and efforts could prove challenging as their many efforts unfold in response to the ever-changing needs of their local communities. Of all education providers, community colleges are arguably the most engaged with the public workforce system.

Community colleges work with various local, regional, state, and federal agencies to establish and expand workforce training programs. These programs exist in degree, certificate, and nondegree forms. They range in completion time from a few weeks to two years and typically closely associate with local employer demands. More and more, community colleges are embracing apprenticeship programs that provide simultaneous pathways to education attainment and employment. These efforts are supported by the community college's mission to increase access to education for all; thus, the colleges remain open-enrollment institutions—meaning all students who apply will gain admission. Accepting students from all socioeconomic and academic preparedness levels creates challenges. These challenges emphasize the criticality of the connection between the community college system and the public workforce development system.

Current statistics help to illustrate the need for partnerships between the two systems. According to the Georgetown University Center on Education and the Workforce (2020), 70% of all jobs will require at least some education beyond secondary schooling by 2027. Expectations suggest the demand for "some college and no degree" workers will decrease as technology and automation change required tasks within occupations. As all sectors of the economy automate, the basic skills required to obtain entry-level employment increase. Local community colleges should and must excel at providing training and education of required competencies aligned with the needs of local employers.

While the public workforce system serves a wide range of individuals, it often does not align with the education system and proves cumbersome and confusing for users to navigate. To effectively educate and train our nation's future workers, community leaders and policymakers must work to understand and align systems and related funding to support lifelong learning while ensuring the existing system remains responsive and flexible. Workforce training efforts are primarily national in funding, regional in planning, and local in action—and dependent upon holistic planning and partnerships for effectiveness.

Educators, community economic developers, parents, employer representatives, and policymakers should work together to encourage all students to explore available occupations within their region and ensure each understands the educational pathways to specific jobs. Early identification and exposure to potential career interests is a community-wide effort and should not be outsourced to the local secondary or postsecondary system. All regional partners should work together to emphasize efforts to expose and engage both students and dislocated workers with local opportunities. This exposure should occur in various ways, including local industry tours, mock interviews, information sessions, occupation exposure through augmented and virtual reality (AR/VR), videos, and camps on the campus of local community colleges, to name a few. These activities should showcase content and funding. Hosting youth on the community college campuses allows students to immerse themselves in a world they may not otherwise experience.

Career Pathways

One initiative focused on guiding students towards relevant careers is known as the career pathways system. Career pathways are promoted by the U.S. Departments of Labor, Education, and Health and Human Services as a way to encourage better alignment of education, public agencies, and employers. Locally, the pathways align education, training, employment, and human and social services to assist both youth and adults with acquiring related credentials and skills to become work ready (Clagett, 2015). Figure 1 depicts the career pathways.

Figure 1

Integrated Postsecondary Career Pathways

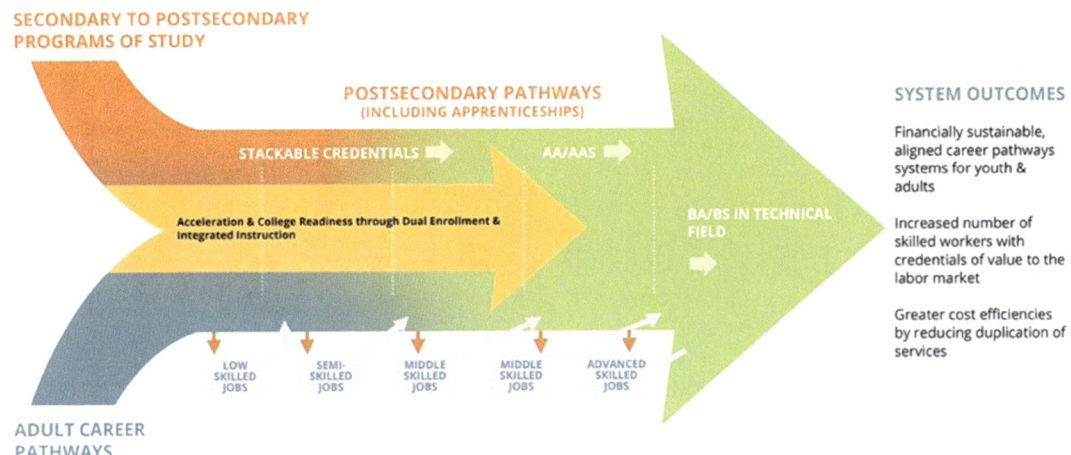

Reprinted from Perkins Collaborative Resource Network (n.d.)

Additionally, formal career pathways enable community economic developers to understand their role in the operation of the local education and training ecosystem. Industry, community economic development entities, and local leaders should support local pathway initiatives. These stakeholders often guide workforce efforts to specific needs such as new training programs, enhanced curricula, and customized training for employers—thus remaining vital in establishing quality career pathway development guidance.

Local leaders should partner with secondary education providers to encourage students to prepare for postsecondary education and training or entry to the labor market upon graduation. Long pathways impede success. Students need to understand available options and the ability to "hop off" their pathway when life circumstances require it. Students also need to be shown where they can "hop on" once they are ready to reenter the workforce preparation path. To make any real progress toward a pipeline of labor market success, the community's focus at the secondary and postsecondary levels must center on preparing high school graduates for whichever path they choose—entering the workforce immediately following graduation or continuing their education and further developing their human capital.

Human Capital Trends

New regional patterns of growth and decline emerged between 2008 and 2017, according to the United States Department of Agriculture (USDA, 2019). Nonmetro counties across the country experienced population decline. In fact, 16 out of 23 states that previously experienced growth during the 2001–2008 time frame lost population between 2010 and 2017. Recreation areas and retirement destinations such as the Pacific Coast, the Ozarks, the Gulf of Mexico, and the southern Atlantic Coast experienced rapid growth in population. Additionally, nonmetro counties near large and medium-sized metro areas continued to experience growth. These communities, like those near Atlanta, Georgia; Raleigh–Durham, North Carolina; and Minneapolis–St. Paul, Minnesota, continued to show a growth rate greater than 5 percent. Rural America was not as fortunate; most nonmetro and farming counties across the country, including those within the Appalachian region, experienced population loss.

The shifting population is of particular importance as a region's human capital becomes more important to winning new economic development projects. Community economic developers and companies evaluating potential sites understand these data points and whether a specific region is likely to grow or shrink. While it may not appear all positive, knowing the realities of a community can enable community leaders to increase its marketability. More importantly, this information can help align leaders and stakeholder community expectations. It will also keep communities from wasting time and valuable resources required to chase opportunities that are not a match. Changing demographics should be monitored here as well. Many nonmetro farming and manufacturing towns report aging populations while metro regions experience an influx of younger populations. This remains an important element in matching communities with development opportunities.

Community and economic developers must understand their local and regional workforce pipeline and how it relates to a region's *laborshed*. A laborshed is the area from which an employment center draws its commuting workers (Iowa, 2017). Communities often support a workforce from outside of their direct governmental boundaries. Understanding where workers live can help a community identify the future pipeline, relevant training partners, and additional types of companies the community may consider recruiting based on the skills and competencies existing within the laborshed. Another term used in economic development is available labor. Many times, companies will examine the laborshed to determine the type and quantity of available labor; these studies are typically performed off concentric rings showing various miles or minutes required to travel to the proposed worksite. Understanding and communicating where a community's labor derives from may improve development opportunities if those findings differ from the data available to companies reviewing communities.

As populations age and shift and as new technologies appear, workforce training initiatives shift as well. In some regions, manufacturing serves the communities as the largest employer; in others, healthcare or government serves this role. Regardless, the skills required continue to change. While workforce training typically occurs within community college facilities, community economic developers must be mindful of these changes and engage in efforts to expose younger students to the technologies present in their local communities.

Partnering for a Skilled Workforce

The workforce pipeline continues gaining importance for economic development projects. As the emphasis shifts from analyzing the local labor market to ensuring that a steady stream of skilled workers exists, communities must closely examine stakeholder interactions. Local, regional, and state partners should coordinate activities, funding, and marketing to best encourage a holistic workforce ecosystem in which residents are aware of opportunities and available resources. Effective partnerships for workforce development are collaborative and support the needs of local employers. While educating and training the workforce pipeline is the responsibility of the education partners, other stakeholders—local employer partners, elected officials, and community leaders—must provide guidance, feedback, and policy assistance to accomplish goals beneficial to all partners. Additionally, local partners must understand and coordinate with regional and state partners to enable the full breadth of opportunities for the local ecosystem.

Employer partners must remain mindful that education's business cycle lasts longer than that of most industries—typically a semester (four months) as opposed to 30 days. Community colleges receive scrutiny regarding their ability to provide a steady pipeline of workers for potential companies. Employer partners may assist secondary and postsecondary partners in highlighting available occupations for which to encourage students to pursue technical training. Many community colleges cite enrollment as the biggest challenge facing their future. As employers demand more skilled workers, community colleges struggle to fill programs; the challenge is clearly a disconnect within the pipeline. Additionally, many employers create alternative pathways into jobs, which effectively compete with the efforts of local training partners. Partners should work to uncover these challenges and find solutions that positively impact the community and the long-term ability to recruit students to and through training programs to ensure a steady pipeline of skilled workers. The public workforce system and career technical funders continuously increase the importance of creating partnerships, leveraging funding, and braiding funds where feasible to ensure populations in need have the ability to access resources.

Funding Public Workforce Development Efforts

Funding workforce development efforts comes in many forms and through many national, state, and local agencies and organizations. Community economic developers should consider developing an asset map to identify local, regional, and state funding agencies if one is not available. Local community college and job center leaders can assist in this effort. Further, while community economic developers may not need to be experts in the funding specifics, they would benefit from an awareness and general understanding of basic provisions of two pieces of key legislation: the Workforce Innovation and Opportunity Act and the Strengthening Career and Technical Education for the 21st Century Act.

Workforce Innovation and Opportunity Act (WIOA)

The Workforce Innovation and Opportunity Act (WIOA) became law on July 22, 2014. It replaced the Workforce Investment Act (WIA) of 1998 and amended the Adult Education and Family Literacy Act, the Wagner-Peyser Act, and the Rehabilitation Act of 1973. WIOA serves to assist jobseekers and vulnerable populations in accessing employment, education, training, and supportive services needed for success. WIOA authorizes programs administered through the Department of Labor to assist adults, dislocated workers, and youth through grants to states. Additionally, WIOA authorizes family literacy programs and state vocational rehabilitation services, which are administered by the Department of Education. WIOA is the latest legislation regarding the public workforce development system and focuses efforts on improving the system to serve clients. Many local activities are guided by WIOA requirements. As such, community economic developers may not need to be experts on such legislation; understanding the basic tenants below, however, may provide a more well-rounded approach to workforce development.

- **Strategically aligned state workforce development programs:** Every state must submit a four-year strategic plan to meet the workforce needs of employers.

Employment and training services are required to be complementary and coordinated so jobseekers acquire skills, credentials, and experience meeting employers' needs.

- **Increased accountability:** Core programs must report on common performance indicators, measure effectiveness of services, and ensure results are made publicly available.

- **Improved promotion of work-based training:** The workforce system is designed to be demand-driven to match employers with skilled individuals. Funds may be used to meet employers' needs through incumbent worker training, transitional jobs, on-the-job training, customized training, and registered apprenticeships.

- **Increased investments in serving vulnerable populations:** Individuals with disabilities, vulnerable youth, Native American populations, and migrant and seasonal farmworkers receive access to high quality workforce services designed to prepare them for competitive employment.

- **Strengthened workforce development boards:** States have various methods for establishing their workforce boards; however, WIOA requires them to coordinate and align programs to serve clients and ensure the board is made up of representatives primarily from employers to guide programs.

Strengthening Career and Technical Education for the 21st Century Act

The Strengthening Career and Technical Education for the 21st Century Act (Perkins V) became law on July 31, 2018. Perkins V serves as the reauthorization of the Carl D. Perkins Career and Technical Education Act of 2006 (Perkins IV) and represents the chance to expand opportunities for students to explore career technical occupation pathways. Key features of Perkins V include:

- supports secondary and postsecondary training programs through funding;

- promotes the development of activities integrating academic, career, and technical instruction, including linking secondary and postsecondary education for participating CTE students;

- increases flexibility for states and local areas to provide services;

- supports secondary, postsecondary, local workforce investment boards, business and industry, and intermediary partnerships; and

- increases employment opportunities for special populations.

Perkins V serves the workforce pipeline by funding career technical education training parallel to WIOA. While there are many more funding mechanisms, establishing a baseline knowledge of Perkins V and WIOA is vital to the success of the workforce ecosystem and integral to developing a comprehensive approach to improving a region's human capital.

Workforce Development Plan

While many agencies engage in the funding and operation of workforce development efforts, too frequently leaders make observations as opposed to getting involved with the process and driving results. Often, leaders and members quickly identify challenges, concerns, and issues with various activities or results within their own communities but cannot identify assets or solutions. Working together to develop an action plan related to workforce development may assist all involved in recognizing the assets within the community many remain unaware of. To develop this plan, community economic developers could:

- identify all local, regional, and state partners and related literature, policy, and relevant labor market data;

- host workforce strategy sessions to allow for brainstorming activities to encourage creativity, involvement, and buy-in;

- develop an asset map with stakeholders identifying current training providers, current funding sources, and available labor;

- identify workforce needs of local employers through focus groups, surveys, or one-on-one meetings;

- work with the broader community to establish a vision for the community's labor market, which may be accomplished during other community development visioning sessions as well;

- develop an action plan in partnership with the broader community to address any skill or provider gaps (This plan should operate in coordination with the region's economic development plan to allow for coordinated recruiting and staffing efforts. Additionally, the plan should include all relevant data and analysis to ensure the plan is demand- and data-driven);

- establish an annual evaluation plan, including related metrics;

- communicate the results, plan, and evaluation mechanism to the broader community and allow for feedback;

- use data to guide holistic workforce programs, services, and activities designed to lead the community to the desired future;

- commit to an awareness campaign to build knowledge of available resources, occupations, and educational options leading to good jobs

A workforce development plan can take many forms and have many uses. Each state has a state plan that should be referenced in local actions. Additionally, many of the processes and strategies taught related to physical infrastructure development can be employed to encourage human capital development.

A community's human capital serves as one of its most valuable assets, but efforts to skill, reskill, and upskill must be part of a good community development plan. Developing partnerships and plans to positively influence the development of the workforce pipeline should be on every community economic developer's to-do list if not already accomplished. While the skills needed shift within the marketplace and may change over time, solid partnerships lead to prepared communities and workforce ecosystems.

Case Study
FlexFactor: Technology Sector Outreach and Recruitment

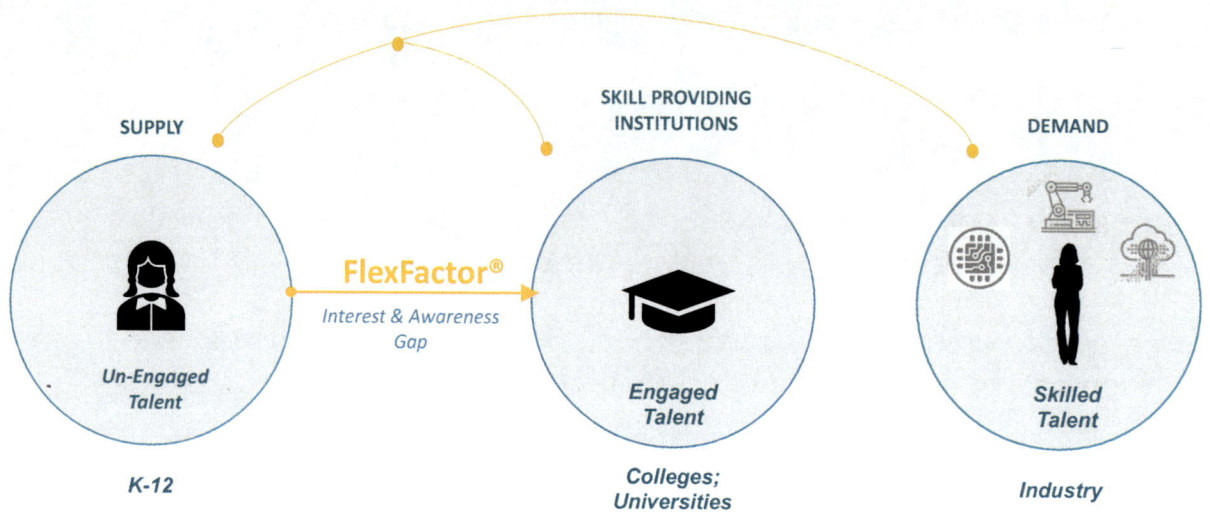

One of the frequently overlooked barriers to workforce development for the STEM sector is the interest and awareness gap. Recognizing this, NextFlex, a Manufacturing USA Innovation Institute with a focus on domestic advanced manufacturing, created FlexFactor.

FlexFactor is an outreach program designed to recruit students into STEM sector education and career pathways. By collaborating with partners from K–12, higher education, and industry, the program engages students with advanced technologies, entrepreneurship concepts, and STEM sector careers. Using a project-based learning framework, FlexFactor challenges small teams of students to identify a real-world problem, conceptualize an advanced hardware product to address it, build a business model around the product, and pitch it to a panel of industry representatives. Through the program, students visit an advanced manufacturing facility to discover how technologies are used and engage with engineers working in the field; they also tour a community college campus to learn about the educational pathways that lead to the jobs they observed during the industry tour. Through FlexFactor's applied approach to learning, students become interested in STEM-based pathways by learning how technical skills solve real-world problems they care about.

FlexFactor's unique immersive framework provides community colleges with a powerful tool to directly engage and recruit students from their K–12 feeder districts, focusing particularly on those pathways most sought after by industry partners. This hands-on relationship building also ensures high school students have the awareness, orientation, and support to build two-year and CTE pathways into their education and career plans.

Through this innovative combination of experiential learning and educational orientation, FlexFactor introduces diverse groups of students to opportunities in the advanced manufacturing field. To learn more, visit https://www.nextflex.us/learning-programs/flexfactor/.

References

Benhabib, J. & Spiegel M.M. (1994). The role of human capital in economic development: Evidence from aggregate cross-country data. *Journal of Monetary Economics. 34*(2), pp. 143–173. https://doi.org/10.1016/0304-3932(94)90047-7

Blum, E.S. & Shepelwich, S. (2017). Engaging workforce development: A framework for meeting CRA obligations. Federal Reserve Bank of Dallas. https://econpapers.repec.org/bookchap/fipfeddmo/00005.htm

Carnevale, A.P, Stroh, J. & Gulish, A. (2015). *College is just the beginning: Employers' role in the $1.1 trillion post-secondary education and training system.* Center on Education and the Workforce, Georgetown University. https://cew.georgetown.edu/wp-content/uploads/2015/02/Trillion-Dollar-Training-System-.pdf

Clagett, M.G. (2015). *Advancing career and technical education (CTE) in state and local career pathways project:* Final report. Office of Career, Technical and Adult, Education, U.S. Department of Education. http://s3.amazonaws.com/PCRN/docs/AdvCTEFinalReport012816.pdf

Conway, M. (2011, August 1). Where labor supply meets labor demand: Connecting workforce development to economic development in local labor markets. Aspen Institute. http://www.aspenwsi.org/resource/update6/.

Georgetown University Center on Education and the Workforce. (2020). The overlooked value of certificates and associate's degrees: What students need to know before they go to college. https://cew.georgetown.edu/cew-reports/subba/.

Iowa Workforce Development. (2017). State of Iowa laborshed analysis: The stats: Job search resources. https://www.iowaworkforcedevelopment.gov/laborshed-studies.

Mikelson, K.S. & Nightingale, D.S. (2004). Estimating public and private expenditures on occupational training in the United States. United States Department of Labor. https://wdr.doleta.gov/research/FullText_Documents/Estimating%20Public%20and%20Private%20Expenditures%20on%20Occupational%20Training%20in%20the%20United%20States.pdf

National Skills Coalition (2020). *Skills mismatch: Lack of access to skills training hurts workers and businesses.* https://nationalskillscoalition.org/resources/publications/middle-skill-fact-sheets/file/US_skillsmismatch.pdf

Nightingale, D.S. & Eyster, L. (2018). Results and returns from public investments in employment. In S. Andreason, T. Greene, H. Prince & C.E. Van Horn (Eds.). *Investing in America's workforce: Improving outcomes for workers and employers*, p. 99. W.E. Upjohn Institute for Employment Research.

Perkins Collaborative Resource Network. (n.d.) *Career pathways system.* https://cte.ed.gov/initiatives/career-pathways-systems

U.S. Department of Agriculture (USDA). (2019). *Shifting geography of population change.* https://www.ers.usda.gov/topics/rural-economy-population/population-migration/shifting-geography-of-population-change/

U.S. Department of Labor. (n.d.) *Wagner-Peyser Act employment service results.* https://www.doleta.gov/regs/statutes/wag-peys.cfm

Wright, P. & McMahan, G. (2011). Exploring human capital: Putting "human" back into strategic human resource management. *Human Resource Management Journal 21*, pp. 93–104. https://onlinelibrary.wiley.com/doi/abs/10.1111/j.1748-8583.2010.00165.x

Made in the USA
Las Vegas, NV
18 December 2023